PRENTICE-HALL
FOUNDATIONS OF IMMUNOLOGY SERIES

EDITORS

Abraham G. Osler

*The Public Health Research Institute of the City of New York
and New York University School of Medicine*

Leon Weiss

The Johns Hopkins University School of Medicine

THE
IMMUNE SYSTEM
OF
SECRETIONS

THOMAS B. TOMASI, JR., M.D., Ph.D.
Mayo Medical School

PRENTICE-HALL, INC., *Englewood Cliffs, N.J.*

Library of Congress Cataloging in Publication Data

TOMASI, THOMAS B   date
    The immune system of secretions.

    (Prentice-Hall foundations of immunology series)
    Includes bibliographies and index.
    1. Immune response.   2. Immunoglobulins.
3. Secretion.   I. Title.   [DNLM: 1. Mucous membrane—Immunology.   2. Mucous membrane—Secretion.
3. Immunity.   QW563 T655i]
QR186.T65   599'.02'9   75-42000
ISBN   0-13-451609-5

10   9   8   7   6   5   4   3   2   1

PRINTED IN THE UNITED STATES OF AMERICA

PRENTICE-HALL INTERNATIONAL, INC., *London*
PRENTICE-HALL OF AUSTRALIA PTY. LIMITED, *Sydney*
PRENTICE-HALL OF CANADA, LTD., *Toronto*
PRENTICE-HALL OF INDIA PRIVATE LIMITED, *New Delhi*
PRENTICE-HALL OF JAPAN, INC., *Tokyo*
PRENTICE-HALL OF SOUTHEAST ASIA PTE. LTD., *Singapore*

To

Roy P. Forster, William van B. Robertson, and Robert F. Loeb,
inspiring teachers who were instrumental in the development
of my early biological and medical foundations,

AND TO

Henry Kunkel, a superb scientist whose help, encouragement,
and friendship engenders a deep sense of gratitude and
admiration.

Foundations of Immunology Series

This series of monographs is intended to provide readers of diverse backgrounds with an authoritative and clear statement concerning significant aspects of immunology. Each volume represents an individual contribution by a distinguished scientist. As a series, they provide a comprehensive view of the field.

The editors have encouraged the individuality of each author in content and method of presentation. They have sought as the major objective of the series, that each monograph be comprehensible and of interest to a broad audience. The authors provide an authoritative treatment of important problems in major research areas, in which rapid development of new information requires an integrated and reliable evaluation. The series should therefore prove valuable to advanced college students, graduate students, medical students and house staff, practitioners of medicine, laboratory scientists, and teachers.

ABRAHAM G. OSLER
LEON WEISS

Contents

Preface

This monograph will deal with an area of immunology concerned with immune reactions occurring locally at mucous membrane sites. Although studies reporting differences between "systemic" versus "local" immunity have appeared in the literature for a number of years, the potential importance of these differences has only recently come into focus. The book attempts to summarize the current data available concerning the concept of local mucosal immunity and to indicate the chemical and biological basis for this concept. The secretory or mucosal system is now recognized as having unique characteristics, particularly the predominance of IgA type antibodies, and is thought to play a key role as a first line of defense against invasion by potentially pathogenic microorganisms and viruses. As a result, techniques of immunization against both bacteria and viruses have recently focused on attempts to elicit high concentrations of antibody in fluids that bathe the mucosal membranes which represent the portal of entry of many microorganisms. In some cases, immunization appears to be most effective when performed by local application of antigens such as aerosolization, whereas in others, depending on the antigen, large doses administered systemically may be the best method of achieving high concentrations of antibodies at the level of the mucous membrane. When systemic immunization is used to produce mucosal immunity, the majority of evidence suggests that the antigen reaches the mucosal sites and elicits locally produced (largely IgA type) antibodies. However, some apparent exceptions occur where transudation of antibodies (largely IgG) from serum may be important in mucosal protection.

An area that has only recently been investigated is the role of local cell-mediated immunity in the mucosal system. The evidence is already substantial that cell-mediated reactions can be elicited in the respiratory tract against several organisms quite independently of systemic cellular immunity. Local immunity mediated by T cells and/or macrophages may be important both in protection of the mucous membrane from colonization and in the complex process of recovery from infections.

The finding that prior immunization affects the absorption of antigens from the gastrointestinal tract has implications in terms of the normal regulation of absorption of macromolecules. These findings also raise the possibility that defects in the mucosal system, particularly in the respiratory and gastrointestinal tracts, may lead to the entrance of antigens normally excluded by immune reactions. The absorbed antigens could elicit the production of antibodies in systemic lymphoid tissues (spleen, lymph nodes) which are cross-reactive with self-antigens and/or form immune complexes, thus leading to the possibility of so-called autoimmune syndromes. In fact, the frequent association of autoimmunity, particularly lupus-like syndromes, with IgA deficiency and the description of patients with circulating immune complexes consisting of milk protein antigens suggest that further studies in this area may be of considerable importance.

THOMAS B. TOMASI, JR.

Rochester, Minnesota

Chapter 1

Introduction and Historical Aspects

The scientific discipline now designated as immunology had its origins in studies pertaining to the mechanism of resistance to infection. It has been known since the pioneering work of Pasteur that following recovery from certain infectious diseases there appears an increased resistance to reinfection which is specific for the organism involved. During the early days of immunology there was much discussion and debate concerning the mechanism of this immune state, and several opposing schools arose. One of these, headed by the Russian zoologist E. Metchnikoff, attributed immunity to the cells of the reticuloendothelial system, while the other, championed by Paul Ehrlich, believed that circulating substances called antibodies were primarily involved. We now know that both mechanisms are operative in varying degrees in the immune response to different agents. For example, it is well established that the rejection of foreign skin or other organ transplants is mediated largely by cellular immunity, while the lysis of red blood cells that occurs following a transfusion reaction is due primarily to serum antibodies directed against the incompatible red blood cells. In many instances, for example in resistance to certain infectious diseases, both cellular and circulating antibody responses occur. In these cases it seems probable that both mechanisms are involved in resistance to, as well as recovery from, infections, although the relative importance of each is not always known.

Until relatively recently, much more emphasis has been placed in immune reactions on the antibodies which are found in the circulation. Almost all of the knowledge available concerning the chemistry of interactions of antibodies with antigens, as well as the more recent information on the structure of the antibody molecule, has been derived from studies utilizing serum antibody. Moreover, in studies on the efficiency of immunization, serum titers of antibodies are usually taken as a primary measure of the effectiveness of the immunizing antigen. Indeed, in many cases there appears to be an excellent correlation between the titers of antibodies against the immunizing agent (for example, a killed bacteria or virus) and the resistance of the immunized individual to reinfection. However, this is not always found and, as will be shown in more detail in a subsequent chapter, resistance to infection with certain organisms is not well correlated with the titer of serum antibody.

The lack of correlation between serum titers of antibodies and resistance to infections was also noted by earlier workers. In 1919, primarily as a result of experimental studies on oral infections with toxin-producing enterobacteria and skin infections with Bacillus anthracis, Besredka postulated that local immunity could be established independently of circulating antibody and systemic immunity. In 1927, he published a now classical manuscript, "Local Immunization," which summarized the evidence available at that time suggesting that a regional immune state could exist without significant participation from serum antibody. Subsequently, additional observations extended the concept of local immunity. Particularly important was the work of Burrows and his co-workers on experimental cholera in guinea pigs, and of Fazekas de St. Groth on influenza virus infection in mice. Burrows clearly showed that resistance to the cholera organism in the guinea pig model was primarily mediated by antibodies present in the gastrointestinal secretions, which he called coproantibody. Since this organism does not invade beyond the mucous membrane and causes its disease primarily by producing an exotoxin in the lumen of the bowel, it seems reasonable that effective immunity must be mediated by antibody present on or near the mucous membrane. The origins of the coproantibodies were not elucidated by Burrows, but some evidence was presented that they may not be derived from serum, at least by simple transudation. This is illustrated in Fig. 1–1 by the temporal dissociation of fecal and serum agglutinins following immunization and by the effects of irradiation. The serum antibody titers are much more radiosensitive than are fecal agglutinins.

In the early 1950s, Fazekas de St. Groth showed that in the respiratory tract, resistance to experimental infection with the influenza virus seemed to be directly related to the content of antibody in the fluids bathing the mucous membrane. If antibody was present in these fluids in significant titer, it prevented the implantation of the influenza virus which, like cholera, is a superficial infection localized to the mucosa.

Older studies in veterinary medicine also suggested local antibody formation in the reproductive tract of several animal species. The literature on these findings has been extensively reviewed by Pierce and has involved primarily the three major infectious diseases causing infertility in cattle (trichomoniasis, vibriosis, and brucellosis). Immunity to these diseases, besides its theoretical interest, is of considerable economic importance. As Pierce points out in his review, it is common knowledge in veterinary medicine that the presence of antibodies to these organisms in vaginal secretions is a more reliable index of infection in the herd than are the titers of the same antibodies in serum. Moreover, in some cases, it is possible to demon-

(a)

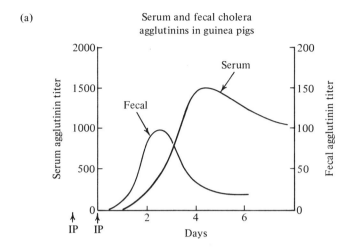

(b)

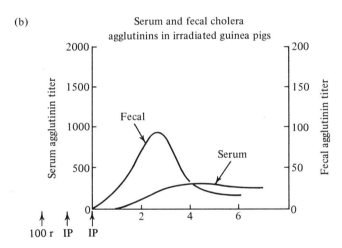

Fig. 1-1. (a) Serum and fecal cholera agglutinins in guinea pigs following systemic (intraperitoneal IP) immunization. (b) Similar studies in irradiated guinea pigs. These studies illustrate the independence of serum and secretory antibodies. (Data redrawn from W. Burrows et al., *J. Inf. Disease,* 87:158, 1950), and M. Koshland et al., *J. Immunol.,* 65:93, 1950.)

strate that local immunization with the killed vaccine will result in the appearance of significant titers in vaginal fluids with little or no serum antibody. On the other hand, parenteral administration with the same antigen produces high titers of circulating antibody with very little antibody in either the vaginal, cervical, or uterine secretions.

Needless to say, these studies, and others of more recent vintage which will be reviewed in detail later, suggest that with certain infections, local immunity rather than circulating antibody may be of primary importance in resistance and defense.

In spite of the observations mentioned above, the concept of local immunity and the full implications of these findings were not fully appreciated until basic information became available concerning the structure of the antibodies present in mucous secretions. Since the description of the chemistry of the secretory antibodies in 1965, there has been renewed interest in the type of biological studies performed by Fazekas de St. Groth and others in the early fifties. Their practical application to immunization against a variety of infectious diseases in man is now apparent.

The groundwork necessary for the characterization of the secretory antibody molecules was laid by studies in the mid fifties and early sixties, which defined the heterogeneity of the serum antibody molecules. These studies clearly showed that antibodies occurred in a variety of different classes, subclasses, and genetic types which differed not only in their chemical structure but in biological properties. Most important was the description of the IgA class of antibodies by Heremans in 1959, since this class of antibody appears to predominate in most secretions. In 1963, it was discovered by Tomasi that a number of mucoantibodies were not only primarily of the IgA class, but that they differed in their chemical and biological properties from the IgA which is found in serum. Muco- or secretory antibodies were shown to be predominantly formed in lymphoid-plasma cells which lie in intimate anatomical relationship to the mucous membrane epithelium. Thus, the phenomenon of local immunity apparently depends on the local production of specific antibody probably synthesized in large part in response to transmucosally absorbed antigens. These considerations have led to the concept that there exists a *secretory immune system* with unique properties which is located in or about the mucous membranes and which in certain circumstances may function quite independently of the *systemic system* which is responsible for the production of circulating antibodies. Although emphasis has focused on the IgA class of antibodies because it is present in secretions in largest amounts, other immunoglobulin classes are also found in external secretions in varying amounts, and evidence is available that, like IgA, they may be produced locally. Moreover, delayed hypersensitivity reactions (cell-mediated immunity) in the respiratory and gastrointestinal tracts have recently been described. Thus, the concept of the secretory system extends to many types of antibodies as well as to cellular immune reactions.

REFERENCES

Besredka, A.: "Local Immunization," Williams & Wilkins, Baltimore, 1927.

Burrows, W., and I. Havens: "Studies on Immunity to Asiatic Cholera. V. The Absorption of Immune Globulin from the Bowel and Its Excretion in the Urine and Feces of Experimental Animals and Human Volunteers," *J. Inf. Dis.*, 82:231, 1948.

Fazekas de St. Groth, S., and M. Donnelley: "Studies in Experimental Immunology of Influenza. III. Antibody Response," *Austr. J. Exp. Biol. Med. Sci.*, 28:45, 1950.

Heremans, J. F., J. P. Vaerman, and C. Vaerman: "Studies on the Immune Globulins of Human Serum. II. A Study of the Distribution of Anti-Brucella and Anti-Diphtheria Antibody Activities Among γss-, γ1M-, and γ1A-globulin Fractions," *J. Immunol.*, 91:11, 1963.

Pierce, A. E.: "Specific Antibodies at Mucous Surfaces," *Vet Rev. Annot.*, 5:17, 1959.

Tomasi, T. B.: "Studies on the Immunoglobulin A Proteins of Serum and Nonvascular Fluids," thesis, Rockefeller University, New York, 1965.

Tomasi, T. B., and S. Zigelbaum: "The Selective Occurrence of γ1A Globulins in Certain Body Fluids," *J. Clin. Invest.*, 42:1552, 1963.

Chapter 2

General Characteristics

of the Secretory Immune System

Originally the concept of a secretory immune system arose as a result of studies in the human indicating that the IgA class of immunoglobulins was the predominant type of antibody present in many external secretions (see the article by Tomasi, Tan, Solomon, and Prendergast in the references at the end of this chapter). These studies, which quantitated the various immunoglobulin classes present in different body fluids, showed a predominance of the IgA class in fluids such as saliva, tears, and the secretions of the respiratory and gastrointestinal tracts. These so-called "external secretions" are all fluids which bathe mucous membrane surfaces, usually with epithelial cells of the cuboidal or columnar type, which are in direct continuity with the external environment. The antibodies present in these fluids are often termed mucoantibodies because of their relation to the mucous membrane. In contrast to external secretions, those body fluids which are contained in closed cavities (internal secretions) do not show the predominance of IgA, and IgG is the major immunoglobulin class. The results of quantitative studies suggested that internal secretions are primarily a transudate from serum and that immunoglobulins occurred in these fluids in proportions determined by molecular size and the permeability of the tissues involved. The concept of internal versus external secretions is presented in Fig. 2–1.

Although IgA is the major immunoglobulin in most external fluids, it is now apparent that the fluids bathing different mucous membranes within the same species vary in their immunoglobulin content. As will be discussed in more detail later, many secretions contain other immunoglobulins, such as IgM and IgE, and these may in large part also be produced locally. To further complicate the picture, there is significant species variation. Although exocrine IgA has been found in all mammals examined so far, in certain cases (e.g., the species bovidae) in addition to IgA, large amounts of IgG are found in colostrum and milk and this is selectively transported from serum. Despite these complicating features there are certain common char-

6

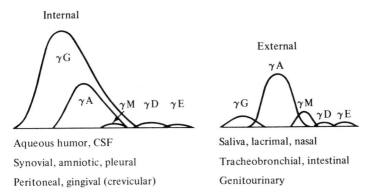

Fig. 2-1. Secretions characterized by immunoglobulin content. The relative concentrations of the various immunoglobulin classes in external and internal secretions are proportional to the areas under the curves.

acteristics of the secretory system which suggest that it can be considered as a distinct entity. First is the presence in external fluids of the various immunoglobulin classes in proportions significantly different from those in serum, and second is the apparent independent regulation of serum and secretory antibody content by either local synthesis and/or selective transport. Biologically these phenomena are of considerable importance since they may lead, under conditions of natural infections as well as immunization, to dissociation between systemic and local mucous membrane immunity.

Immunoglobulin Content
of Various Human Secretions

Significant technical difficulties are encountered in the quantitation of the various immunoglobulins in secretions. Each secretion is a complex mixture of proteins and other constituents, some of which appear to be derived from serum and others produced locally by the mucous membrane or glandular epithelium. The problems of analysis vary from secretion to secretion. For example, with bile some of the pigments are extremely difficult to remove and therefore interfere with the colorimetric reactions commonly used to measure proteins. Nevertheless, using specific antisera, it has been possible to at least roughly estimate the proportions of the various immunoglobulins present in these fluids. For the most part, data are available only for the three major immunoglobulins, IgA, IgG, and IgM. IgE and IgD are present in secretions in very small amounts and are difficult to measure, although recently some data have become available on the IgE content of a few secretions.

It is beyond the scope of this book to discuss all of the various technical problems involved in the quantitation of immunoglobulins in secretions. However, since quantitation is of such key importance to the concept of the secretory system, a brief review of some of the major difficulties seems appropriate. For more detail, the reader is referred to several recent articles by Tomasi and Bienenstock, and by Brandtzaeg, listed at the end of this chapter.

Perhaps the most commonly used technique for quantitating immunoglobulins in biological fluids is the radial diffusion method described by Mancini. This method involves incorporating a specific antiserum directed against a given immunoglobulin class into agar and placing a measured amount of the test fluid in a small hole cut in the agar. Following a precise period of incubation, measurement is made of the diameter of the ring of precipitation formed as the antigen diffuses into the antibody-containing agar. The diameter of the ring, compared to that produced by standards of known concentration, is then a measure of the concentration of the antigen (immunoglobulin) in the test fluid. However, since the size of the precipitin ring depends also on the rate of diffusion (diffusion coefficient) of the antigen, this technique is extremely sensitive to antigen size. It is necessary, therefore, to use a standard immunoglobulin preparation of the same size as that in the test fluid. For example, in the quantitation of IgA in saliva containing predominantly 11S IgA, if a 7S IgA standard isolated from serum is used, the amount of IgA will be underestimated approximately threefold. Since most secretions contain mixtures of different sizes of IgA, it is difficult to devise an appropriate standard and the values obtained are therefore only approximations. Another significant problem is that exocrine secretions often contain immunologically reactive fragments of IgG and IgM which are smaller than the native molecules. Their presence can lead to an overestimate of the concentration of the immunoglobulins if the native proteins are used as standards.

In some cases, particularly with IgD and IgE, the Mancini technique is not sensitive enough to detect immunoglobulins in unconcentrated secretions. Therefore, concentration is necessary and this may be attended by considerable losses. An alternative technique, electroimmunodiffusion, is sensitive enough to be used directly on unconcentrated fluids, but has the same disadvantage in regard to polymers and fragments as does radial diffusion. In this technique, antibodies are also incorporated into the agar, but electrophoresis is carried out prior to immune diffusion. Other techniques such as quantitative precipitation and complement fixation which are not as dependent upon molecular size have been used, but they either lack sufficient sensitivity (precipitation) or are interfered with (complement fixation) by other nonimmunoglobulin substances present in some external secretions. The double-antibody test is one of the better techniques for measuring small quantities (as little as 10 ng/ml) of immunoglobulin (Ig) in secretions. In this technique, radiolabelled I^{131} Ig is interacted with anti-Ig and the complex precipitated with an anti-antibody (Coombs reagent). The ability of the test fluid to inhibit precipitation of the label is proportional to its Ig concentration. This technique is capable of measuring IgE in unconcentrated saliva or nasal wash fluids.

Quantitation of immunoglobulins in secretions such as those of the gastrointestinal tract and bile are complicated by additional problems. Proteolytic enzymes present in these fluids may degrade immunoglobulins. There are also substances in these secretions which give a nonspecific precipitation with goat and other animal sera. These latter reactions are nonimmune and are due to electrostatic interaction between an unknown component(s) present in these secretions and an alpha globulin in the antisera. Such nonspecific reactions can often be avoided by isolation of the antibody containing (gammaglobulin) fraction from the immune sera.

In some cases it is difficult to obtain "native" secretions because of the limited amounts of these fluids available in the normal state. For example, it is necessary to stimulate the flow of tears with an irritating substance, and nasal and bronchial fluids are usually obtained by irrigation of the mucous membrane. Therefore, the values reported for immunoglobulin concentrations and antibody titers in these fluids frequently do not apply to the native secretions.

In most reports the concentration of an immunoglobulin or other components is expressed as milligrams per milliliter of secretion. However, with certain fluids the concentrations may change significantly with flow rate. For example, the IgA concentration of parotid fluid is three to four times lower in stimulated versus nonstimulated saliva. However, the actual rate of secretion of IgA (i.e., micrograms of IgA per minute) may increase three- to fourfold on stimulation. Thus, it would be difficult to compare data from different reports on IgA concentration in parotid saliva unless the rates of secretion were known. It is preferable, therefore, in the case of the saliva to express concentrations of immunoglobulins in terms of secretory rates. Similar reasoning applies to urine where flow rates and immunoglobulin concentrations may change in opposite directions.

Overt inflammation in a secretory organ can significantly change the proportion of the various immunoglobulins present in the secretion of that organ. This frequently results from transudation of proteins from serum since increases in local capillary permeability are a well-known consequence of inflammation. In addition, there may be an invasion of the site by inflammatory cells from the outside (circulation), particularly by cells producing IgG, and this may significantly alter the relative proportions of cells producing the various immunoglobulin classes. In certain tissues the normal, or at least the customary, situation is one of a low-grade inflammation. In the newborn or in animals which are kept in a relatively germ-free state, one sees very few immunoglobulin-producing cells in the gastro-intestinal and respiratory tracts. As these sites become colonized by micro-organisms and antigens are ingested and inhaled, immunoglobulin-pro-ducing cells begin to appear. Thus, one could argue that in many tissues of the secretory system there exists a "physiological inflammation." The degree of this inflammation and therefore the immunoglobulin content may vary considerably in different individuals, races, and geographic locations. For example, it has been shown that there exists a good correlation between the extent of periodontal inflammation about the teeth and the content of IgG and IgM in whole saliva. Thus the concentrations of the immuno-globulins in saliva are significantly affected by dental status. Similarly, it might be expected that in tropical areas where parasitic and bacterial infection in the GI tract are common, the normal immunoglobulin content of the GI secretions might differ from those found in this country.

Considering the difficulties mentioned above and emphasizing the ap-proximate nature of the values obtained, some data on the immunoglobulin content of various secretions are recorded in Table 2-1. The values were

Table 2-1

The content of immunoglobulins in external fluids and numbers of lymphoid-plasma cells in the corresponding mucous membrane. The number of cells containing the different immunoglobulins were determined using the fluorescent antibody technique.

Organ or secretion	Concentration of immunoglobulins (mgm%)			Concentration ratio	Cell count ratio
	IgG	IgA	IgM	IgG/IgA	IgG/IgA
Serum	1,000	160	100	6	—
Colostrum	10	1,234	61	0.008	—
Breast milk [a]	30	600	50	0.05	—
Parotid	0.03	10	0.04	0.003	1:50
Whole saliva	7	37	0.8	0.2	—
Nasal [b]	10	20	0–Tr	0.5	1:6
Lacrimal (tears)	0–Tr	20	—	<0.1	1:12
Bronchial [b]	20	28	—	0.7	1:5
Gastric	—	—	—	—	1:16
Duodenum	10	31	21	0.3	—
Jejunum	34	28	—	1.2	1:22
Ileum	30	35	—	0.9	—
Colon	86	83	—	1	1:23
Rectum	—	—	—	—	1:16
Appendix	—	—	—	—	1:1
Gallbladder (bile)	143	160	—	0.9	—

[a] Average value in first three days. Concentration of all immunoglobulins falls as lactation proceeds.

[b] Fluids obtained by irrigation of nasal mucosa and tracheobronchial tree.

obtained immunologically using specific antisera and the Mancini technique described above. The standard used in the radial diffusion technique was an 11S IgA molecule isolated from colostrum. Data on the relative numbers of IgA versus IgG cells obtained by the fluorescent antibody technique on the corresponding tissues are included.

Many external secretions contain, in addition to the 11S species, higher polymers of secretory IgA (15–20S) and also significant amounts of 7S IgA. For example, human parotid saliva contains approximately 10% 7S IgA, whereas small intestinal fluids have about 35% 7S IgA. The relative proportions of the various sizes of IgA are usually determined by fractionation on Sephadex G-200 or by sucrose density gradient ultracentrifugation. It is difficult to determine whether the higher polymers are normally present or at least partly produced during the fractionation procedure. The 7S IgA in some secretions such as saliva is mostly derived from serum. This can be shown by injecting I^{131}-labelled IgA intravenously and then analyzing the saliva for the distribution of radioactivity by density gradient ultracentrifugation. However, in other fluids such as colostrum and GI secretions, much more 7S IgA is present than can be accounted for by simple transudation, and it seems likely that it is either secreted as such or results from depolymerization of 11S IgA subsequent to secretion.

The IgG present in secretions appears to be very similar if not identical to that present in serum, both in immunological as well as physicochemical properties. A large part of the IgM in saliva is complexed to secretory component. In some cases, particularly in gastrointestinal fluids, Fab and Fc fragments of IgG and IgM are also detected. These probably result from proteolysis since the majority of secretory fluids contain proteolytic enzymes. An exception is parotid fluid which does not have detectable proteolytic activity. In addition to the three major immunoglobulins, IgD and IgE can also be detected in some secretions, but in very small amounts. For this reason there is a paucity of quantitative data available on these immunoglobulins. IgD has been detected in saliva and GI fluids, and IgE in urine, tears, nasal fluids, and saliva. Very few physicochemical studies have been done on these immunoglobulins. In one report, salivary IgE was found to be very similar or identical to serum IgE in size and antigenic characteristics.

QUANTITATION OF SECRETORY COMPONENT IN BIOLOGICAL FLUIDS

Recently, because of the availability of antisera which react specifically with the unbound or free form of secretory component (SC) (see Chapter 3), it has become possible to quantitate the amount of free secretory component (FSC) in various biological fluids. Normal human unstimulated parotid saliva contains approximately 3.0 mg% of FSC and about 209 mg% is present in colostrum. Since SC represents about 15% of the secretory IgA molecule by weight, it can be calculated that about 50% of the SC in parotid saliva is bound in secretory IgA, and about 50% is free. Similarly, approximately 50% of the SC is bound to IgA in whole human colostrum. Patients with agammaglobulinemia or individuals who have a selective deficiency of IgA have approximately normal amounts of FSC in their saliva.

Using antisera specific for the secretory component, it has been found that SC determinants can be detected by gel precipitation in normal sera. By Sephadex G-200 chromatography and density gradient ultracentrifugation, it was demonstrated that serum SC was attached to IgA and that all normal human sera contained very small amounts of circulating secretory IgA (about 0.005 mg/ml). Markedly elevated levels of secretory IgA (SIgA) are seen in certain diseases which involve the mucous membranes such as enterocolitis and chest infections. Some of the highest levels approaching 0.2 mg/ml are found in lactating women. One could postulate that these elevated levels are due to release or "backflow" of SIgA into the serum in conditions involving inflammations of the mucous membranes. However, this is not always the case, since high levels of serum SIgA are also seen in disorders such as rheumatoid arthritis and multiple myeloma in which there is no known involvement of the mucous surfaces. It is interesting that the concentration of SIgA in human cord serum, although lower in absolute amount than in normal adult serum, comprises about 40% of the total IgA. Animal sera have not been extensively studied for SIgA. There is one report in which bovine serum was found to contain 0.065 mg/ml of SIgA, which represents about 20% of the total serum IgA of that species.

REFERENCES

Brandtzaeg, P.: "Human Secretory Immunoglobulins. IV. Quantitation of Free Secretory Piece," *Acta Path. Microbiol. Scand.*, 79B:189, 1971.

Brandtzaeg, P.: "Local Formation and Transport of Immunoglobulins Related to the Oral Cavity," in *Host Resistance to Commensal Bacteria*, ed. by T. MacPhee, Churchill Livingstone, Edinburgh, 1972.

Tomasi, T. B., and J. Bienenstock: "Secretory Immunoglobulins," in *Advances in Immunology*, ed. by F. Dixon and H. Kunkel, Academic Press, Inc., New York, 1968, p. 1.

Tomasi, T. B., E. M. Tan, and A. Solomon, and R. A. Prendergast: "Characteristics of an Immune System Common to Certain External Secretions," *J. Exp. Med.*, 121:101, 1965.

Chapter 3

Structure of

Secretory Immunoglobulins

GENERAL STRUCTURE OF IgA

The immunoglobulins consist of a complex system of structurally related proteins which are found in the sera of all vertebrates. Their primary physiological role is to mediate antibody activity. The immunoglobulins are unique among animal proteins to the extent to which they show polymorphism. For example, there exists in normal animal serum hundreds of different types of antibodies each with a different primary structure (amino acid sequence). Each of these antibodies presumably arises from a specific stimulus which is triggered by an antigen, and each is more or less specific for the corresponding antigen although cross reactions with compounds other than the stimulating antigen are well known.

The cellular events triggered by antigen and leading to differentiation and proliferation of the antibody producing cells are complex, but it seems very likely that each antibody is produced by a clone of cells, and conversely a single cell produces a single or restricted number of species of antibodies. Modern theories of antibody formation maintain that antigen selects an appropriate and complementary lymphoid precursor cell by reacting with a specific surface receptor which is probably an immunoglobulin. The manner in which specificity for antigen is created is debated. Some workers believe that diversity is in large part inherited in the germ line, others maintaining that somatic mutation plays an important role. With certain antigens, other cell types such as macrophages and thymus-derived cells (T cells) are required in addition to the precursor lymphoid cells (B cells) which bear surface immunoglobulins. The molecular events triggered by antigen which lead to cell differentiation (blast transformation) and proliferation to form a clone of antibody-producing cells are largely unknown.

Despite the great diversity of antibodies, all normal immunoglobulins possess similar overall structural features. The basic unit consists of four

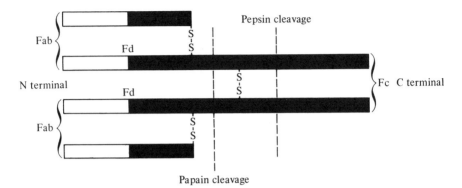

Fig. 3-1. Schematic structure of IgG. The V, or variable, regions of light and heavy chains are open, and the C, or constant, regions are in solid black. The Fc is the crystallizable fragment containing only H chain material; the Fab is the fragment which has the antibody combining site and contains a complete L chain and a portion of the H chain called the Fd fragment. There are two Fab fragments per molecule and therefore two sites that complex with antigen. The number of inter-H-chain disulfides varies in different species and between the subgroups of IgG within a given species.

polypeptide chains: two identical H (heavy) chains and two identical L (light) chains. As illustrated in Fig. 3-1, both the L and H chains have variable (V) and constant (C) regions. Comparison of different antibodies or myeloma proteins of the same immunoglobulin class show very similar amino acid sequence in the C regions, but the V region sequences differ markedly. V and C regions are coded by separate genes and the immunoglobulins are therefore unique in that the synthesis of a single polypeptide chain is controlled by at least two genes. There is substantial evidence that the antibody-combining site is located in the amino terminal portion of the molecule and formed by the cooperative interaction of the V regions of both the H and L chains. It is the marked variability of the V region amino acid sequences that is responsible for the large variety of different combining sites and antibody specificities.

In the majority of immunoglobulins, the L and H chains are covalently linked by disulfide bonds. However, as discussed below, there is a subclass of IgA in which the L and H chains are bonded only by secondary (non-covalent) forces. The L chains are of two types, kappa (κ) and lambda (λ), both having molecular weights of about 22,500, but each having a unique and characteristic sequence of amino acid in their C regions. All normal immunoglobulins have L chains and, in fact, one of the criteria for establishing that a molecule is indeed an immunoglobulin is the presence of L chains. The L chains are primarily, although not solely, responsible for the observed immunological cross reactions between the different classes of immunoglobulins.

It is now recognized that there are five major immunoglobulin classes in the human, and analogous classes have also been described in most other mammalian species. The major classes can be distinguished from one another by physicochemical as well as immunological and biological properties (see Table 3-1). All of the classes share L chains, but each has a dis-

Table 3-1

Properties of different human immunoglobulin classes

	IgG	IgA	IgM	IgD	IgE
Mean serum					
concentration (mgm%)	1,000	160	100	3	0.03
Heavy chain designation	γ	α	μ	δ	ϵ
Sedimentation coefficient	7S	7S(10, 13, 15, 18)	19S	7S	8S
Molecular weight	152,000	160,000	950,000	180,000	200,000
Carbohydrate approx. %	2.5	7.5	10	10	10
Sensitivity to sulfhydryl					
reagents	0	±	+	0	±
T ½	22 [a]	6	5	2.8	2.3
Synthetic rate					
(gm/70 kg/day)	2.3	2.7	0.4	0.03	0.0014
% intravascular	40	40	75	75	50
Placental transfer	+ [b]	0	0	0	0
Association with secretory					
component	0	+	±	0	0
Complement fixation [c]	+	0	+	0	0
Reagin activity	0	0	0	0	+
PCA in guinea pig	+	0	0	0	0
Blocking activity	+	0 [d]	0	0	0
Relative hemagglutinating					
efficiency per μg N	1	2–10	10–25	–	–
Relative hemolytic					
efficiency per μg N	1	0	5–10	0	0
Reaction with rheumatoid					
factor [e]	+	0	0	0	0
Reaches adult levels	1–3 yrs	4–14 yrs	6–12 mos	–	–

[a] T ½ for $IgG_{1, 2}$, and $_4$ subclasses. IgG_3 has mean T ½ of 9 days.
[b] IgG_2 subclass is poorly transported.
[c] References to complement fixation via the classical pathway. IgA and IgE may fix complement via the alternate or C3 shunt pathway.
[d] IgA may have blocking activity in external secretions.
[e] Refers only to classical rheumatoid factor. The sera of multiply transfused, IgA-deficient, and allergic patients may have antigammaglobulin antibodies directed towards other classes.

tinctive H chain which has been given a specific name depending on the class as shown in Table 3-1. In addition to the major classes, subclasses have been recognized. For example, there are four subclasses of IgG in the human and in the mouse. Distinction between a class and a subclass is not always clear since the subclasses are coded by different genes and their H chain constant regions have a unique primary structure. However, subclasses are closely related to one another and probably arose later in evolution from the more primitive class genes. For example, the IgG subclasses all have a C terminal glycine and show extensive homologies in their C regions which are responsible for the cross reactions with certain antisera which characterize them as IgG.

IgA was first isolated and characterized by Heremans in 1959. Its concentration in human serum is relatively small, comprising about 15% of the total immunoglobulins. The relatively low concentration of IgA in human sera is due primarily to its rapid catabolism since the amount of IgA synthesized per day is as great as that of IgG. Thus, considered in terms of daily synthesis, IgA is a major immunoglobulin.

The proportions of kappa and lambda light chains in both serum and secretory IgA are similar to that of IgG, i.e., 60% κ and 40% λ. Using the fluorescent antibody technique, similar proportions of κ and λ light chain containing cells can be visualized in the gastrointestinal tract in humans and in rabbits.

As depicted in Fig. 3-2, two subclasses of IgA have been recognized. The existence of subclasses of IgA was established on the basis of antigenic differences and chemical characteristics such as amino acid sequence and carbohydrate content. For example, the hinge peptide (a short seg-

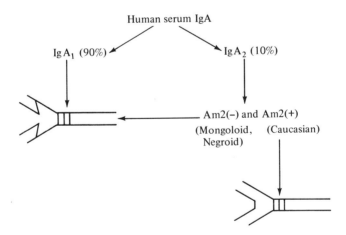

Fig. 3-2. Schematic representation of the human IgA system showing two subclasses (IgA$_1$ and IgA$_2$) and allotypes (Am2($-$) and Am2($+$)). Ninety percent of the serum IgA is IgA$_1$, which has disulfide-bonded H and L chains. Two allotypes of IgA$_2$ exist. The Am2($+$) allotype, which predominates in Caucasians, is composed of L and H chains which are held together by noncovalent bonds; the L and H chains occurring as L-L and H-H dimers.

ment between the Fab and Fc containing the inter-H-chain disulfides) of the IgA$_2$ subclass is nine residues shorter than that of IgA$_1$ and does not contain galactosamine. In fact, the absence of galactose is a marker for the IgA$_2$ molecules. In IgA$_1$ the hinge peptide contains carbohydrate and also has a small segment of seven to eight amino acids which is duplicated in the same region where the IgA$_2$ proteins are deleted (see Fig. 3-3). This

L Chain - - - - Cys

L-H linkage   Ser-Leu-Cys-Ser-Thr-Glx-Pro-Asx.....
                130

Hinge

IgA$_1$ Val-Thr-Val-Pro-Cys-Pro-Val-Pro-Ser-(Thr-Pro-Pro-Thr-Pro-Ser-Pro-Ser)$_2$ -Cys-Cys-His-Pro-Arg

IgA$_2$ Val-Thr-Val-Pro-Cys-Pro-Val-Pro-Pro-Pro-Pro-Pro.................................... Cys-Cys-His-Pro-Arg

C terminal   IgA$_1$ and IgA$_2$ Met-Ala-Glu-Val-Asp-Gly-Thr-Cys-Tyr

               IgM   Met-Ser-Asp-Thr-Ala-Gly-Thr-Cys-Tyr

               IgG   Glu-Lys-Ser-Leu-Ser-Leu-Ser-Pro-Gly

Fig. 3-3. Primary structure of human IgA illustrating several key regions of the molecule. The L-H disulfide linkage occurs at Cys 130 (from N terminus) in IgA$_1$ proteins. This residue may be absent in Am2(+) proteins. The hinge region of IgA$_1$ contains a duplicated segment (enclosed in parentheses) which is depleted in IgA$_2$ (see text). The C terminal octapeptide is identical in IgA$_1$ and IgA$_2$. The C terminal tetrapeptide of IgA is identical to that of IgM and quite different from IgG. (Data from B. Frangione and C. Wolfenstein-Todel, Proc. Nat. Acad. Sci., Washington, 69:3673, 1972; and C. A. Abel and H. M. Grey, Science, 156:1609, 1967.)

suggests that the IgA$_1$ hinge results from the insertion of a partially duplicated gene segment. The function of the hinge region is unknown, but it is possible that the insertion of a short segment of DNA between the duplicated N and C terminal serves to fuse these genes, each of which has specific biological properties, into a single chain.

One of the outstanding features of the IgA$_2$ subclass concerns its disulfide bond structure. Within the IgA$_2$ subclass two allotypes (genetic variants) have been described termed Am2(+) and Am2(−). These genetic variants can be distinguished from one another by the use of appropriate antisera, and IgA myeloma proteins of the IgA$_2$ class belong to either of one of the two allotypes but not both. The outstanding difference between the two allotypes is the absence of the disulfide bonds linking the L and H chains in the Am2(+) variant. Molecules of this type have only secondary forces, probably largely hydrophobic in nature, linking the L and H chains. This may be associated with the absence of the cysteine at position 130 which links the L and H chains in the IgA_1 subclass (although this has not been directly demonstrated), or it could remain as a free SH or intrachain bridge. As depicted in Fig. 3-2, in Am2(+) IgA_2 proteins the L and H chains are present in the molecule as L2 and H2 dimers. It is interesting that the noncovalent forces between the L and H chains are stronger in the Am2(+) molecules than in the IgA_1 or Am2(−) proteins. In Caucasians, the vast majority of the IgA_2 molecules are of the Am2(+) variety; in other populations such as the Mongoloids and Negroids, the Am2(−) allotype predominates. Individuals who receive a foreign allotype in blood transfusions may become immunized against this allotype, and the sera of these individuals therefore contains anti-allotype antibodies. Similarly, IgA-deficient individuals who receive products containing IgA may form antibodies against the IgA (see also Chapter 12).

The majority of mouse myeloma proteins appear to be IgA_2, although myeloma proteins have been described in the NZB strain of mice in which the L and the H chains are disulfide bonded. These may be genetic variants and mice may possess only one subclass corresponding to IgA_2. Relatively little information is available concerning subclasses in other species, but it has been found that the dog, horse, and rabbit all have a proportion of their IgA which has noncovalently bonded L and H chains. Rabbit IgA has been extensively studied, and two subclasses controlled by closely linked loci, each having several allotypic specificities, have been described.

In addition to H and L chains, two other polypeptide chains have been recognized in IgA. One of these chains, secretory component, is present only in the IgA molecule found in external secretions (SIgA). The structure and function of secretory component is discussed in Chapters 2 and 3. The other polypeptide chain, J chain, is found in dimeric serum IgA and IgM in addition to SIgA. J chain is not present in monomeric serum IgA, IgG, IgD, or IgE. This newly described chain may have an important linking or joining function in polymeric immunoglobulins as further discussed later in this chapter.

Amino acid sequence data on a human IgA protein have shown that 55% of the C terminal 40 residues are identical with those of IgM. On the basis of this high degree of homology, it has been proposed that the alpha chain diverged from the μ chain about 175 million years ago (approximately 125 million years after IgG). Since mammals appeared about 175 million years ago, this would place the appearance of IgA very early in mammalian evolution.

In subsequent sections emphasis is placed on the isolation and chemical properties of the IgA in secretions (SIgA). This is because of the paucity of data concerning the structure of immunoglobulins other than secretory IgA, due primarily to their low concentrations in external secretions. It should be emphasized, however, that the biological importance of an immunoglobulin does not necessarily parallel its concentrations. For example, IgE, although present in serum and secretions in small amounts, has important biological functions. From the data presently available, it appears that the IgG and the majority of the IgM and IgE in external secretions have molecular sizes and antigenic properties which are identical to those of their serum counterparts. Several reports have suggested that the relative concentrations of the IgG subgroups may be somewhat different in nasopharyngeal fluids and colostrum than in serum. However, these claims are not well substantiated and accurate quantitation of the IgG subgroups in secretions is not yet available. A relatively large fraction of the IgM molecules (approximately 60%) may contain attached SC. The significance of this finding is not clear, but the observation that the majority of IgM is secreted bound to SC suggests that SC may play an important role in the transport of IgM. However, the majority of IgE appears to be secreted without SC, although a minor species of IgE having a molecular size larger than that of serum IgE (molecular weight 200,000) has been described in saliva. Whether this contains SC or represents aggregates of IgE is not certain.

ISOLATION OF SECRETORY IgA

Homogeneous preparations of SIgA have been isolated from colostrum and milk, parotid saliva, nasal fluids, bronchial secretions, gastrointestinal fluids, and urine. The techniques used to isolate SIgA from these fluids vary both with the fluid and from one laboratory to another, but in general they involve the sequential application of salt fractionation (ammonium sulfate and/or zinc ions), ion exchange chromatography, and gel filtration on Sephadex or Agarose. Colostrum is one of the most convenient starting sources because of its high concentration of IgA. For example, human colostrum (mammary secretions obtained in the first 48 hours) contains from 0.5 to 1.0 gram % of IgA. In other species such as the cow, sheep, and goat, saliva is a good source of SIgA because it is available in large amounts and because it contains smaller amounts of IgG$_1$ which is present in high concentrations in the milk of these species and is difficult to separate from IgA. The purity of the preparations obtained using these procedures is quite variable. Even preparations consistently homogeneous by standard techniques (polyacrylamide gel electrophoresis, analytical ultracentrifugation, and gel diffusion) often contain traces of contaminants which are detected only by the antibody response occurring after immunization of an appropriate animal. The most common contaminant is the iron-containing protein lactoferrin, although other materials such as blood group substances, IgG, and amylase are not uncommon contaminants in SIgA preparations. For more details concerning the isolation of SIgA from various secretions, the reader is referred to several recent reviews by Gally, and Mattioli and Tomasi, listed at the end of this chapter.

CHEMICAL PROPERTIES OF SECRETORY IgA

Some of the physical and chemical properties of SIgA are compared with those of serum IgA and IgG in Table 3-2. The secretory molecule is

Table 3-2

Comparative physical and chemical properties of SIgA

	IgG	IgM	Serum IgA	Secretory IgA
Sedimentation coefficient $s^0_{20,w}$	6.6S	17.9S	6.9S	11.3S
Molecular weight	152,000	950,000	160,000	385,000
Diffusion coefficient $D^0_{20,w}$	4.0	1.75	3.0–3.6	2.43
Partial specific volume, $\bar{v}$	0.740	0.715	0.725	0.717
Frictional ration f/f^0 [a]	1.50	1.92	—	1.75
Extinction coefficient $E^{1\%}_{280m\mu}$	14.3	11.8	13.4	13.9
Molecular weight of H chains [b]	52,000	72,000	58,000	58,000
Carbohydrate %	2.5	7–12	7.5	11.5
hexose	1.1	6.2	3.2	6.2
hexosamine	1.3	3.3	2.3	4.1
fucose	0.2	0.7	0.2	0.7
sialic acid	0.3	1.7	1.8	0.7

[a] Calculated using the Einstein-Smaluchowski and Stokes relationships; $D = kT/f$ and $f^0 = 6h \ (3M\bar{v}/4 \ N)^{1/3}$. See H. K. Schachman, in *Ultracentrifuge in Biochemistry*, Academic Press, Inc., New York, 1959.

[b] Includes carbohydrate.

composed of two 7S IgA monomeric subunits apparently identical to serum 7S IgA, plus an additional nonimmunoglobulin polypeptide chain, secretory component (also called secretory "piece," T chain, or T component). In addition, there is recent evidence, discussed in detail below, which suggests that SIgA contains a fourth polypeptide chain (J chain) which, unlike secretory component (SC), is also found in polymeric serum IgA and IgM. Most of the data in Table 3-2 were obtained on SIgA isolated from saliva or colostrum. However, good evidence is available that the major species of IgA present in other external fluids, including those of the respiratory and gastrointestinal tract as well as urine, are very similar and probably identical to those of salivary and colostral IgA.

The molecular weight (M.W.) of both 11S salivary and colostral IgA is approximately 385,000. One of the major problems in obtaining precise values for the M.W. of SIgA is the lack of accurate data for the partial specific volume, $\bar{v}$, since this quantity is difficult to measure experimentally. In the human, a $\bar{v}$ of 0.723 for SIgA has been calculated from the amino acid and carbohydrate composition of the molecule, while in the rabbit a value of 0.703 has been reported. Assuming that the subunits of the secretory molecule are identical to those of serum IgA and each SIgA molecule contains four light (L) and four heavy (H) polypeptide chains, the expected M.W. of the IgA dimer would be about 312,000 (each L chain with a M.W. of approximately 23,000 and each α chain 55,000). This would leave about 73,000 to accommodate both the SC and J chain. For rabbit SIgA, based on the M.W. of 60,000 reported for the α chain, the calculated M.W. of the IgA dimer would be 346,000. Since a M.W. of 370,000 has been experimentally measured for rabbit secretory IgA, only about 25,000 is available for SC and J chain. This is hardly sufficient since the combined M.W. of these two proteins is approximately 75,000–100,000. The reason for this discrepancy in the rabbit system is not clear, but it seems likely that it may be due to inaccuracies in the determination of the M.W. of the SIgA molecule and/or the α chain. In addition, the possibility exists that the α chains of the SIgA are different from those of serum IgA, although the presently available data are against this.

Salivary and colostral IgA have type κ and λ molecules in about the same ratio as found in serum IgA, i.e., approximately 60% of the SIgA molecule have κ-type and 40% λ-type light chains. This same ratio is also found in the human and rabbit GI tracts when cells containing κ and λ determinants are counted using the fluorescent antibody technique. The vast majority of intestinal lamina propria cells contain either κ or λ determinants but not both, similar to the findings in peripheral lymphoid tissues. Thus, although each cell of the secretory system possesses the genes enabling it to synthesize both classes of L chains, the final antibody-producing cell (plasma cell) synthesizes only one gene product.

IgA$_1$ and IgA$_2$ subclasses are both represented in colostral and salivary SIgA, although the relative amount of the IgA$_2$ type appears to be greater than in serum. For example, it has been found that human milk may contain as much as 30–50% of the IgA$_2$, whereas this subclass constitutes only about 10% of serum IgA. No special function has been attributed to either of these subclasses so that the significance of the increased proportion of IgA$_2$ in certain secretions is undetermined. However, as will be discussed later in this chapter, the IgA$_2$ in human milk (SIgA$_2$) is unique in that, unlike its serum counterpart, the L and H chains appear to be covalently bonded. This may create a stabilizing influence so that SIgA$_2$ molecules do not dissociate in denaturing conditions. This could provide a selective advantage for antibodies functioning in the hostile environment found on mucous surfaces.

When treated with proteolytic enzymes in vitro, SIgA is more resistant to degradation than is serum IgA or IgG. The evidence for this statement stems from experiments in which the degree of degradation of SIgA is compared with serum IgA and IgG following incubation with crystalline proteolytic enzymes such as trypsin, chymotrypsin, or pepsin or with intestinal juice. Reasoning teleologically, this relative resistance to proteolysis could represent a biological advantage for SIgA antibodies which function in complex secretions containing proteolytic activity. However, resistance is only relative and some proteolysis does occur. It has been possible, using pepsin and trypsin, to isolate 5.0S F(ab)$_2$-like and 3.5S Fab-like fragments.

Intact Fc fragments are not produced from the human SIgA molecule by these enzymes, although papain and trypsin both give rise to Fc-like fragments containing SC from rabbit SIgA. A new enzyme, called IgA protease, has recently been isolated from cultures of streptococcus sanguis, which produces good yields of an Fc fragment from human IgA. This enzyme is highly specific for IgA and does not proteolyze IgG, IgM, or other nonimmunoglobulin substrates such as casein and hemoglobin. It can also be isolated from human colonic secretions and may play an important, although presently undefined, role in the ecology of the secretory system. Two subclasses of rabbit SIgA have been described by antigenic analysis, f and g. The f subclass is resistant to cleavage by papain, whereas the g molecules are split into Fab and Fc fragments. The structural differences between the two subclasses have not yet been fully identified. Naturally occurring Fc-like fragments are also found in normal human feces (perhaps produced by IgA protease) and in the serum and secretions of patients with α chain disease (see Chapter 12 for a discussion of α chain disease).

On treatment of 11S human SIgA with disulfide bond reducing agents (0.01 M dithiothreitol or 0.1 M β-mercaptoethanol), no evidence of dissociation occurs on subsequent analytical ultracentrifugation. In this respect the secretory molecule is quite different from polymeric serum IgA which, under similar conditions, dissociates completely into 7S subunits. This observation forms the basis for the often-quoted statement that human SIgA appears to be more resistant to dissociation with sulfhydryl reagents than its serum counterpart. However, these findings should not be taken to indicate that disulfide bonds have not been split in SIgA since the addition of small concentrations of urea (2 molar) following reduction will cause dissociation. Thus, it appears that under mild conditions of reduction, some disulfide bonds in SIgA are cleaved but the molecule is held together by noncovalent forces. This can be shown in vitro by reconstitution of the 11S IgA molecule following simple incubation of 7S serum IgA with reduced-alkylated SC. Since the sulfhydryl groups in SC are blocked, reconstitution apparently depends on noncovalent associations. By careful reduction and alkylation followed by gel filtration, it has been possible to obtain subunits of human SIgA which correspond to 7S IgA. In addition, a few molecules are obtained which appear to be formed by two α chains bound to SC.

ISOLATION AND CHEMICAL PROPERTIES OF SECRETORY COMPONENT

Several methods are available for the isolation of SC. Originally, SC was obtained by reduction and alkylation of SIgA isolated from colostrum or saliva. Following reduction, chromatography is performed on Sephadex G-100 in 0.5 N propionic or acetic acid. The distribution of SC in the eluate is tested immunologically using SC specific antisera. Those fractions containing SC but not L chains are pooled and rechromatographed on Sephadex G-200 in aqueous buffers. Preparations of SC obtained by this method are often contaminated with small amounts of other components particularly lactoferrin and α chains. Recently SC has also been isolated in the free form from colostrum and saliva. The procedures used to isolate free SC (FSC) have varied, but one of the most satisfactory involves precipitation of colostral whey with 50% ammonium sulfate, followed by DEAE chromatography and gel filtration on Sephadex G-200. Similar procedures have been applied to the isolation of FSC from bovine colostral whey and milk. The bovine FSC is considerably easier to obtain in homogenous form than human FSC. The secretions of patients with agammaglobulinemia or with a selective deficiency of IgA can be used to advantage since FSC is present in these fluids and isolation is somewhat easier because of the absence of immunoglobulins.

Some of the chemical properties of human SC are outlined in Table 3-3. It should be noted that the molecular weight of the human SC isolated by reduction and alkylation of the human colostral IgA molecule and determined in the ultracentrifuge is on the order of 60,000 while that obtained for FSC by gel filtration or polyacrylamide SDS gels is 75,000–

Table 3-3

Properties of human secretory component

Sedimentation coefficient $s^0_{20,w}$	4.2S
Molecular weight:	
sedimentation equilibrium	58,000–72,000
gel filtration and SDS gels	75,000–85,000
Carbohydrate %	9–12
Unique amino acid composition	High glycine, No methionine

85,000. The possibility exists that the SC molecule is altered somewhat by reduction and alkylation. Alternatively, perhaps as a result of some unusual characteristic of the molecule such as molecular asymmetry or charge distribution, the values obtained by the sieving techniques are abnormally high. Similar molecular weights have been obtained for both bovine and rabbit SC. In all three species, SC appears to be a single polypeptide chain. A previous report suggesting that SC consisted of two polypeptide units of approximately 25,000 each appears to be in error since the authors were probably dealing with the rabbit J chain rather than SC. Rabbit and bovine SIgA, like the human, have additional antigenic determinants not present on serum IgA, and these determinants have also been identified on the polypeptide chains which occur free in secretions and which have certain properties (M. W. and cross-species binding to IgA) similar to human SC. In the case of the bovine secretory component, analogy with the human has been demonstrated by the finding that 13 out of the first 15 N terminal amino acid residues in the SC of the two species are identical.

It is most important to recognize that SC is not an immunoglobulin, and studies thus far do not suggest a relationship between SC and L or H chains. The evidence for this statement stems from the following observations. SC has a distinctive amino acid composition (high glycine, no methionine) which is different from that of H or L chains. Unlike immunoglobulin chains, it is produced in epithelial rather than lymphoid plasma cells and is present (without immunoglobulins) in the secretions of newborns and agammaglobulinemics. Finally, recent sequence studies on the bovine SC have shown no amino acid homology in the first 15 residues with either L or H chains. However, more complete sequences for the human protein are needed to determine if some more distant but significant relationship occurs between SC and H and/or L chains.

Secretory component is probably bonded to the α chain in the SIgA molecule. The evidence for this is as follows:

1. SC complexes with IgA and not to other immunoglobulins. Since the various classes share L chains and have unique H chains, the specific binding of SC to IgA presumably resides in its H chain.

2. In patients with α chain disease, an Fc-like fragment of the α chain has been identified in their saliva and this contains covalently bound SC.

Using rabbit SIgA it has been possible to produce with papain and trypsin an Fc fragment which has covalently bound SC. Using a newly described enzyme, IgA protease (see above), human SIgA yields an Fc fragment containing SC.

Evidence suggests that the linkage of SC in human SIgA involves two types of forces: approximately 80% of the molecules contain SC bonded by both covalent (disulfide) and noncovalent forces. In the remaining

599.029 591 m
c. 1

20%, SC is bonded solely by noncovalent or secondary forces. This is suggested by the observation that approximately 15–20% of the SC can be dissociated from the IgA portion of the SIgA molecule by chromatography in the presence of agents such as acid or 8M urea which inhibit secondary forces. In the rabbit, a significantly larger fraction of the SC is linked by noncovalent forces, since about 60–70% can be dissociated with urea alone; the remaining 30–40% appears to be bonded by disulfide bonds in addition to secondary forces.

In Vitro Binding of SC to Serum Proteins

Binding studies employing I^{131}-labelled human SC and human proteins show specificity of in vitro complexing of reduced-alkylated SC and FSC for IgA. In these studies, FSC was labelled with I^{131} and incubated with whole serum or isolated immunoglobulin preparations. Binding was measured either by immunoelectrophoresis followed by autoradiography (Fig. 3-4) or in some cases by shifts in the distribution of the radioactive SC on Sephadex gel filtration as demonstrated in Fig. 3-5. It was clearly shown that SC binds specifically to the IgA_1 and IgA_2 subclasses but not to other serum proteins. An exception is a small amount of binding with IgM. In one series of experiments, it was shown that FSC derived either from human

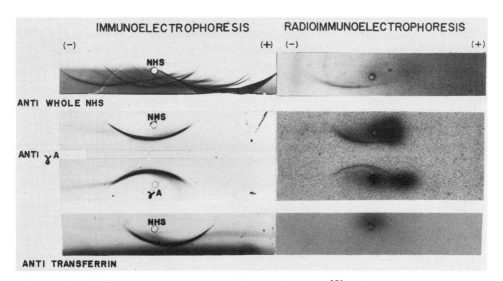

Fig. 3-4. Radiolabelling experiments showing specific complexing of I^{131}-labelled secretory component with serum IgA (γA). Complexing does not occur with IgG, IgM, transferrin, or other serum proteins. Stained immunoelectrophoretic patterns on left, corresponding radioautographs on right. (NHS = normal human serum.)

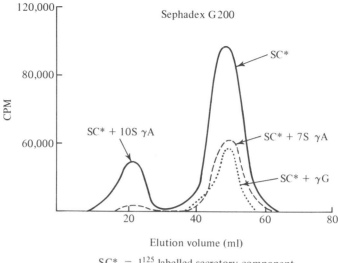

$SC^* = I^{125}$ labelled secretory component

Fig. 3-5. Sephadex G 200 chromatograph of in vitro mixtures of radiolabelled bovine secretory component (SC) with human IgG, 7S IgA, and 10S IgA. Note that the 10S IgA complexes significantly with SC, as shown by the appearance of radioactivity in the void volume when SC and 10S IgA are incubated before chromatography. A small amount of binding of SC to 7S IgA may also occur.

or bovine milk would specifically bind with the serum IgA's of nine different mammalian species. Rather surprising in these studies was the fact that the binding of bovine FSC was quantitatively similar for each of the species studied. Thus, binding of SC seems to be a unique property of IgA and may be a useful ancillary method of identifying IgA in various mammalian sera.

An interesting and potentially important observation is the specificity of binding of bovine FSC for polymeric IgA. This is most dramatically shown using polymer and monomer human myeloma IgA isolated from the same serum. Binding is selective for the polymer. Unexpectedly, it was found that after simple in vitro incubation, binding of FSC was primarily by covalent bonds. Thus, it appears that SC readily participates in disulfide interchange reactions with IgA and to a lesser extent IgM, but not with other serum proteins. A similar interchange reaction occurring in vivo could be responsible for the formation of SIgA from the 10S IgA dimer and SC at the mucosal level.

As discussed earlier the Am2(+) genetic variant of human IgA_2 lacks disulfide bonds between the L and the H chains and the protein can be dissociated by denaturing solvents such as acid, urea, or detergents into L_2 and H_2 dimers. When an isolated 10S IgA_2 Am2(+) human myeloma protein is incubated in vitro for 1 hour at 37°C with either human or bovine SC, the protein becomes stabilized. This is evidenced by the inability of denaturing solvents such as 1M propionic acid, urea, or detergents which inhibit secondary forces to dissociate the reconstituted SIgA molecule. Since stabilization is prevented by iodoacetamide which blocks disulfide interchange, it seems likely that stabilization results from the formation of disulfide bridges. In this respect, the action of SC is similar to certain disulfide interchange enzymes which have been described in mammalian tissues.

Since dimeric IgA contains J chain, it has been suggested that the specificity of binding of the bovine FSC for the polymer is determined by the presence of J chain in the molecule either directly or indirectly through some conformational effect. However, this appears unlikely for the following reasons. Although bovine FSC shows specificity for the polymer, human FSC is capable of complexing with monomeric Am2(+) human myeloma proteins. It is also found that bovine FSC prevents the release by detergent of L chain dimers from F(ab')2a fragments produced by pepsin proteolysis of IgA. Since both monomer IgA and F(ab')2a fragments do not contain J chain, it is obvious that the in vitro binding does not require the presence of this polypeptide chain. This is shown in Fig. 3-6, which also demonstrates that the products of this reaction are consistent with a covalent complex consisting of one molecule of SC and one F(ab')$_2$a. The ability of human SC to complex with monomer IgA may explain the observation that a small percentage of the 7S IgA in human colostrum does contain SC. However, since there is a considerable quantity of FSC in human milk, it might be expected that an interaction with 7S IgA leading to complex formation would occur and that the majority of 7S IgA in colostrum and milk would possess attached SC. It is pos-

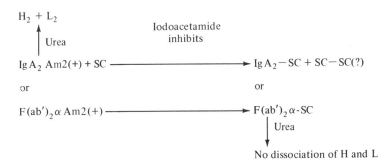

Fig. 3-6. Postulated reaction mechanisms in the stabilization of IgA by secretory component (SC). Incubation of myeloma proteins of the IgA$_2$ subclass (or their F(ab')$_2$ fragments) with SC produces IgA molecules which fail to dissociate H and L dimers on treatment with urea. Since the reaction is inhibited by iodoacetamide, a disulfide interchange mechanism is postulated.

sible that the bulk of the 7S IgA in human milk is of the IgA_1 subclass, and it has been found that the human FSC binds only to monomer IgA_2, Am2(+) proteins, and not 7S IgA_1 or with the monomer IgA_2 Am2(−) genetic variant (L. M. Jerry, personal communication).

The above observations are consistent with and perhaps an explanation for the observation that, when isolated preparations of human colostral SIgA derived from individuals who are Am2(+) are subjected to poly-acrylamide electrophoresis in 0.1% sodium dodecyl sulfate, very small amounts of L_2 dimers are released despite the fact that 30–50% of the total SIgA is of the IgA_2 Am2(+) subclass (see Fig. 3-7). This suggests that stabilization of the L-H bonds by SC is a naturally occurring phe-

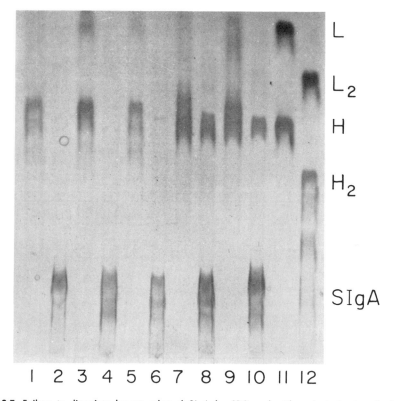

Fig. 3-7. Failure to dissociate human colostral SIgA by SDS-acrylamide gel electrophoresis. The five samples of SIgA in the even-numbered wells from 2 to 10 fail to release a light chain dimer (L_2) band in detergent. Yet in the alternate odd-numbered wells heavy (H) and light (L) chains are released after partial reduction and alkylation, as seen best in wells 3, 7, and 9. An IgA_2 myeloma protein marks the position of H_2 and L_2 in well 12, and after partial reduction and alkylation, H and L in well 11. The SIgA samples in wells 8 and 10 are contaminated with albumin which migrates close to the H chain position. (Data from L. M. Jerry, H. G. Kunkel, and L. Adams, J. Immunol., 109:275, 1974.)

nomenon. It has been suggested that such stabilization may enhance the capacity of the IgA_2-type antibodies to function in the hostile environment found in secretions. If further studies do in fact substantiate this view, then the relative enrichment in the IgA_2 subclass found in certain secretions may be a result of selective pressures developed during evolution.

As noted before, the cysteine residue at position 130 from the N terminus which links the L and H chains in the IgA_1 subclass may be missing in the IgA_2 Am2(+) myeloma proteins, although this has not been established. If Cys 130 is indeed deleted, then the stabilization which results from SC binding to IgA_2 proteins does not involve the formation of the same L-H disulfide linkage as found in native IgA_1 and IgA_2 Am2(−) proteins. The exact position of the disulfide bonds induced by SC and the mechanisms involved are the subject of current investigations in several laboratories.

CHEMICAL PROPERTIES OF J CHAIN

In 1970 Halpern and Koshland reported that rabbit SIgA contained an additional polypeptide chain unrelated to L or H chains or SC. This component, referred to as J (for joining) chain, was first noted as an anodally fast migrating component in urea polyacrylamide gels following the complete reduction of SIgA which had previously been stripped of SC by treatment with urea. A similarly fast migrating component has been identified in SIgA, polymeric serum IgA, and IgM in several species including the mouse, dog, rabbit, and human. J chain bands, usually two to four in number, have been identified in urea polyacrylamide gels in human polymeric serum IgA, SIgA, and IgM, but not in monomeric IgA, IgG, or IgE. Convincing evidence for the existence of this component as a structural part of the IgA molecule is the finding that J chain is present only in polymeric IgA and not in the 7S monomer derived from the serum of the same myeloma patient. This is illustrated in Fig. 3-8. J chain is not found in either the Fab or $F(ab)_2$ fragments derived from IgM and IgA. Positive gel precipitin reactions with J chain antisera and IgM Fc preparations have been reported, suggesting localization of J chain in the Fc fragment of IgM. However, the specificity of the antisera has been difficult to define. This is because generally the anti-J antisera are weak and it is difficult to exclude a reaction with a μ or α chain fragment of about the same size as J chain which has been produced by prior proteolysis of the IgA or IgM protein. In this regard, it is very common to find evidence of some proteolysis in preparation of IgM and IgA myeloma proteins. In fact, some evidence suggests that these proteins may bind proteolytic enzymes such as plasmin, and this could be responsible for the often observed release

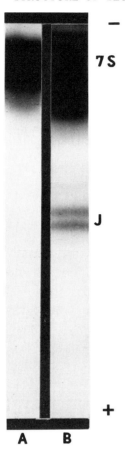

Fig. 3-8. Polyacrylamide gel electrophoresis in 8M urea. Reduced and alkylated monomer (gel A) and polymer (gel B) of the same IgA myeloma protein. Note J chain in polymer but not monomer IgA.

of proteolytic fragments from the isolated proteins following reduction of their disulfide bridges. Recently C terminal sequence studies have shown that J chain is bonded to the penultimate cysteine on the H chain of IgA and IgM.

J chain can be isolated from polymeric IgA or IgM by any one of a number of reported methods. Usually the L and H chains are first separated by reduction and alkylation followed by chromatography on Sephadex G-100 in a dissociating buffer such as 4M guanidine. Under these conditions, the J chain is contained within the L chain peak. The L-J mixture is then separated by one of several techniques which include preparative polyacrylamide electrophoresis, ion-exchange chromatography, anti-L-chain immunoadsorbent, or dialysis against distilled water.

J chain has been estimated to have a molecular weight from 15,000 to 30,000 daltons with the higher molecular weights being obtained on SDS polyacrylamide gels. A molecular weight of about 18,000 for human

J chain has been obtained in our laboratory by equilibrium ultracentrifugation. It contains approximately 8% carbohydrate which includes hexose, hexosamine, and sialic acid. J chain has been isolated from the rabbit, dog, and human SIgA molecules and shown to have a very similar amino acid composition. One noteworthy characteristic of J chain is the high content of the amino acid cysteine (six to eight half-cystine residues) compared to L chains (five half-cystine residues). The marked similarity in the amino acid composition between the J chains from different species may be responsible for the difficulty that is frequently encountered in producing strong antisera against J chain, i.e., the number of species-specific antigen determinants on the J chain may be quite small. This is also suggested by the marked similarity in the electrophoretic mobility and banding patterns of J chains from various species on polyacrylamide gel electrophoresis. For example, the mobility of the J chain derived from the shark 19S IgM is very similar to that of human and other mammalian species. Sharks are among the earliest vertebrates having an immune system arising in evolution about 300 million years ago, before the divergence of the various immunoglobulin classes. They have a single immunoglobulin class which occurs in antigenically identical 19S and 7S forms, closely resembling IgM in their properties. The 19S IgM like proteins contain J chain, while the low molecular weight (7S) IgM does not. These findings suggest that J chain arose early in evolution and has probably undergone relatively few evolutionary changes in its structure.

One of the key questions concerning the J chain which arose early after its discovery concerns the possibility that it is not a unique polypeptide chain but rather a fragment derived from either the L or H chain. That the J chain is a separate polypeptide chain is suggested by the following observations: (1) The amino acid composition of J chain is quite different from that of either L or H chain. (2) The N terminal peptide isolated after pronase digestion of J chain has an amino acid composition different from that found in any H or L chain studied thus far. (3) The amino acid composition of the cysteine-containing peptides isolated from the J chain are quite different than those of the L or H chain derived from the same molecule. In these experiments, a human IgA myeloma protein was reduced and alkylated with C^{14} iodoacetamide. J chain was then separated from H and L chains, digested with trypsin and pepsin, and the cysteine (radiolabelled) peptides isolated by paper electrophoresis. Their amino acid composition was then determined and compared with the cysteine peptides isolated from the H and L chains. (4) The marked similarities in chemical properties and the immunological identity of the J chain isolated from human IgA and IgM. If J chain were a fragment of the heavy chain, it would be expected that the J chain derived from IgA and IgM would show more differences than have been thus far observed. (5) The absence of J chain in the IgA monomer when it is present in the polymer of the same myeloma protein makes a fragment of the α or L chain unlikely. (6) Antigenically, J chain has been reported to be quite different from either H or L chain; however, as mentioned above, the specificities of the J chain antisera have not been rigorously proven. Although accurate quantitative data are not yet available from the yields of J chain obtained from IgA and IgM, it appears that there is a single J chain per molecule of dimeric IgA and 19S IgM.

By immunofluorescence, J chain is found in the same cells (lymphoid-plasma cells) as IgA and IgM. Synthesis of J chain has also been demonstrated using in vitro culture techniques in cell lines derived from mouse myeloma that produce polymer IgA or IgM but not those that produce only monomer IgA. Analysis of intracellular versus extracellular IgA in mouse myeloma cells has shown that, although the majority of intracellular IgA is monomeric, a significant proportion (about 20%) is polymeric and only the latter contains J chain. This has been interpreted as indicating that polymerization and complexing with J chain are late phenomena occurring just prior to the exit of the IgA from the cell, perhaps on or near the surface membrane. Complex formation with J chain may be catalyzed by a disulfide interchange enzyme.

Since both monomer and polymer IgA proteins occur in normal as well as in human and mouse myeloma sera, it is necessary to postulate either that only certain cells produce J chain or, alternatively, that J chain is produced in all IgA- and IgM-producing cells, but for unknown reasons, only a fraction of the molecules combine with it and consequently polymerize. The IgA monomer-polymer ratios characteristic of various species could be determined by the availability of J chain. For example, in the human, where the majority of serum IgA is 7S, only limited amounts of J chain may be available; other species such as the dog would have sufficient J chain to polymerize essentially all of their IgA. Another possibility is that two types of cells exist, one synthesizing monomer without J chain, the other J chain and polymeric IgA. However, in the myeloma system both the monomer and polymer are presumably products of a single clone of cells, and it is difficult to visualize the origin of two cell types differing in their ability to synthesize J chain.

The biological significance of J chain is as yet unknown. Because its presence is restricted to polymeric immunoglobulins such as IgA and IgM, it has been suggested that it is involved in linking or joining their subunits. However, experiments designed to demonstrate such a role have been conflicting; some workers report that J chain is necessary for the assembly of 7S IgM monomers to the 19S pentameric form, while others have found that J chain was not required for reassociation of the IgM subunits. Recent experiments in the author's laboratory have pro-

vided some evidence that in IgM J chain may be involved in the intersubunit linkage. In these experiments, monoclonal 19S IgM proteins were
reduced under mild conditions (0.02 M β-mercaptoethylamine) which are
known to selectively cleave the intersubunit disulfide linkages. These conditions result in the formation of about 30% 7S IgM. After alkylation, the
19S IgM was separated from the 7S IgM by Sephadex G-200 chromatography. Bands with a mobility consistent with J chain were found in the light
(2S) region of the chromatograph. Analysis of the 7S fractions by polyacrylamide electrophoresis in 8M urea indicated that there was no significant dissociation of the molecules into L and H chains and, therefore, only
the intersubunit bonds had been cleaved. The isolated 19S and 7S fractions
were then more vigorously reduced (0.05 M dithiothreitol) in order to
release any residual J chain. J chain bonds were found only in the 19S and
not in the 7S IgM fractions. These studies indicate that J chain is released
under conditions which selectively split intersubunit bonds and suggest
that J chain is involved in the intersubunit linkage. Analysis of the IgM
system has shown that with mild reducing conditions it is possible to produce a noncovalently bonded pentamer. In this species, the J chain appears
to link two 7S IgM subunits but the remaining three are noncovalently
bonded. In the native (unreduced) molecule there may be two types of
disulfide bonds, those involving J chain and those in which the subunits
are directly complexed to each other without J chain. I have hypothesized
that the role of J chain is to produce a conformational change in the IgM
subunits which induces noncovalent interactions, and that these in turn
allow close apposition of SH groups on adjacent subunits and, therefore,
disulfide bond formation. Similarly, in the IgA system, Dr. Stephen Hauptman and I have found that the IgA dimer containing J chain is the most
stable unit. Higher polymers of IgA, when mildly reduced, dissociate into a
stable dimer (with J) and IgA monomers (without J). Elegant quantitative
studies of disulfide chemistry of IgA and IgM from Dr. Koshland's laboratory have led to similar conclusions (see the article by Chapuis and
Koshland listed at the end of this chapter). A hypothetical model for the
formation of an IgA polymer is illustrated in Fig. 3-9.

Although the studies reviewed above certainly suggest an important
role for J chain, perhaps in joining the subunit of polymeric immunoglobulin molecules, this should be accepted with some caution. It is known
that both IgA and IgM have a propensity to undergo disulfide interchange
reactions with a number of unrelated proteins. For example, about 50%
of IgA myelomas and 75% of monoclonal IgM proteins have covalently
attached albumin. Similarly, a large percentage of IgA myeloma proteins
complex with $\alpha 1$ trypsin inhibitor. These complexes are thought to have
little biological importance, perhaps being formed spuriously during the
process of obtaining the serum. Here again, however, it is possible that

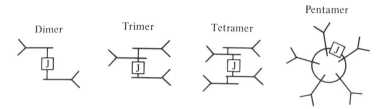

Fig. 3-9. Schematic structure of various-size IgA polymers. The dimer, trimer, and tetramer are depicted as linear molecules as suggested by recent studies (S. Hauptman and T. B. Tomasi, Jr., *J. Biol. Chem.*, 250:3891, 1975) of the disulfide chemistry of IgA polymers. The pentamer of IgA is shown as a circular structure in analogy with the conformation of IgM.

these binding phenomena are of some as yet unknown biological importance. Admittedly, the large number of diverse proteins which complex with IgA suggest nonspecificity, and it is possible that J chain could fit into this category. To this author this seems unlikely, particularly in view of the finding that the vast majority of the IgA and IgM proteins so far examined contain J chain, and unlike most of the other proteins which complex with IgA and IgM, the J chain originates in the same cell as the immunoglobulin. Also important is the finding of J chain in all polymeric molecules of a given protein preparation, suggesting that it is an integral part of the molecule.

THREE-DIMENSIONAL CONFORMATION OF SECRETORY IgA

Relatively little information is available concerning the three-dimensional conformation of secretory immunoglobulins. Some data have been reported on the optical rotatory dispersion (ORD) properties of SIgA. This technique is useful in obtaining information on protein conformation, primarily secondary structure in solution. Immunoglobulins in certain respects are unusual in their ORD behavior. They do not contain significant amounts of α helices, although certain of their optical properties such as a low negative specific rotation suggest the presence of some type of organized structure.

Both serum and secretory IgA are quite similar in their ORD behavior to serum IgG and IgM. Certain organic solvents such as 2-chloroethanol allow nearly optimal conditions for helix formation, and many proteins in this solvent have close to 100% of their residues involved in helix formation. IgG, serum IgA, and 11S SIgA form a maximum of only about 40% helix in 2-chloroethanol, and cleavage of disulfide bonds, in order to remove any possible restrictive influence of this linkage, does not significantly affect their final helical content. The type of structure responsible for the ORD characteristics of the immunoglobulins has not been definitely elucidated, but there is some evidence to suggest the participation of a crossed β-type of conformation. However, the interpretation of conformation of complex proteins such as immunoglobulins from ORD and circular dichroism (CD) spectrums is at present imprecise. It has been postulated that the low helical content of the immunoglobulins is related to the presence in these molecules of large amounts of certain amino acids such as proline, serine, threonine, valine, isoleucine, and cysteine, which do not readily participate in helix formation.

The ORD spectrum of SIgA at lower wavelengths has not been reported. It is known that the small cotton effect at 240 mμ which is typical of IgG is not seen with either IgA$_1$ or IgA$_2$ myeloma proteins, and it would be interesting to determine whether the secretory molecule behaves like serum IgA in this respect. Of note in this regard is the observation that, although native IgA proteins do not show the cotton effect at 240 mμ, their Fab and F(ab')$_2$ fragments clearly show this effect. The observed 240 mμ effect in the native IgA probably results from a larger contribution to the total rotation of the Fc fragment in the whole IgA molecule. No information is available on the CD spectrum of SIgA.

Several electron microscopic techniques have been used to study the architecture of SIgA. Modifications of the conventional negative staining procedures described by Brenner and Horne and of the mica technique have provided improved visualization. In the latter technique, probably due to the capillary forces, molecules tend to stretch out and spread more evenly on the carbon film. As shown in Fig. 3-10, the predominant form is the double ($\succ\!\!\!-\!\!\!\prec$) structures shown fully extended. However, many molecules show a tendency to bending at a point in the middle of the molecules, with angles being observed to vary from 60° to 180° in the completely stretched out molecules. Thus, the SIgA molecule appears to have a high degree of flexibility. The flexibile region in the center of the

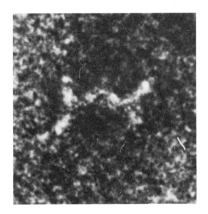

Fig. 3-10. Electronmicroscopic photograph of secretory IgA showing the double Y extended conformation. ✕240,000. (Courtesy of S. E. Svehag, *J. Exp. Med.*, 133:1035, 1971.)

molecule probably represents the joining position of the two monomers. Dimeric serum IgA shows a very similar conformation, including a tendency to bend at the point where the Fc regions join. Therefore, the secretory component could not be clearly visualized by this technique. Upon mild reduction and alkylation, the SIgA yielded single Y-shaped 7S monomers with the dimensions of the Fab 35 × 70 Å and Fc 40 × 70 Å. Mouse myeloma IgA appears to have a similar structure to the human myeloma IgA and SIgA.

R E F E R E N C E S

Chapuis, R. M., and M. E. Koshland: "Mechanism of IgM Polymerization," *Proc. Nat. Acad. Sci.*, 71:657, 1974.

Chuang, C Y., J. D. Capra, and J. M. Kehoe: "Evolutionary Relationship Between Carboxyterminal Region of a Human Alpha Chain and Other Immunoglobulin Heavy Chain Constant Regions," *Nature*, 244:158, 1973.

Frangione, B., and C. Wolfenstein-Todel: "Partial Duplication in the 'Hinge' Region of IgA$_1$ Myeloma Proteins (Amino Acid Sequence/Duplication/Recombination/Gene Fusion/Evolution)," *Proc. Nat. Acad. Sci.*, 69:3673, 1972.

Gally, J. A.: "Structure of Immunoglobulins," in *The Antigens*, ed. by M. Sela, Vol. I, Academic Press, New York, 1973, p. 162.

Halpern, M. S., and M. E. Koshland: "Novel Subunit in Secretory IgA," *Nature*, 228:1276, 1970.

Jerry, L. M., H. G. Kunkel, and L. Adams: "Stabilization of Dissociable IgA$_2$ Proteins by Secretory Component," *J. Immunol.*, 109:275, 1972.

Jerry, L. M., H. G. Kunkel,, and H. M. Grey: "Absence of Disulfide Bonds Linking the Heavy and Light Chains: A Property of a Genetic Variant of γA2 Globulins," *Proc. Nat. Acad. Sci.*, 65:557, 1970.

Kehoe, J. M., C. Y. Chuang, and J D. Capra: "Relation of Carboxyterminal Region of a Human Alpha Chain to Other Immunoglobulin Constant Region Sequences," *Fed. Proc.*, 32:968 (abst.), 1973.

Kobayashi, K., J. P. Vaerman, H. Bazin, A. M. Verheyden, and J. F. Heremans: "Identification of J Chain in Polymeric Immunoglobulins from a Variety of Species by Cross-Reaction with Rabbit Antisera to Human J Chain," *Immunochemistry*, 111:1590, 1973.

Mach, J. P.: "In Vitro Combination of Human and Bovine Free Secretory Component with IgA of Various Species," *Nature*, 228:1278, 1970.

Mattioli, C., and T. B. Tomasi: "The Human Serum Immunoglobulins," *Disease-a-Month,* April, 1970.

Mestecky, J., R. E. Schrohenloher, R. Kulhavy, G. P. Wright, and M. Tomana: "Site of J Chain Attachment to Human Polymeric IgA," *Proc. Nat. Acad. Sci.,* 71:544, 1974.

Plaut, A. G., R. J. Genco, and T. B. Tomasi: "Production of an Fc Fragment from Human Immunoglobulin A by an IgA-Specific Bacterial Protease," in *The Immunoglobulin A System,* ed. by J. Mestecky and A. R. Lawton, Plenum Press, New York, 1974, p. 245.

Tomasi, T. B.: "Production of a Noncovalently Bonded Pentamer of Immunoglobulin M: Relationship to J Chain," *Proc. Nat. Acad. Sci.,* 70:3410, 1973.

Tomasi, T. B.: "Structure and Function of Mucosal Antibodies," *Annual Rev. of Med.,* 11:281, 1970.

Tomasi, T. B., and H. M. Grey: "Structure and Function of Immunoglobulin A," in *Progr. Allergy,* ed. by P. Kallos, and B. Waskman, S. Karger, Basel, 1972, Vol. 16, p. 81.

Wilde, C. E., and M. E. Koshland: "Molecular Size and Shape of the J Chain from Polymeric Immunoglobulins," *Biochemistry,* 12:3218, 1973.

Chapter 4

Immunological Reactions

of Secretory IgA and Secretory Component

When serum and secretory IgA are compared by gel diffusion analysis using antisera made against serum IgA, both molecules appear to be immunologically identical, i.e., they show a reaction of complete identity. Therefore, employing an antiserum made against IgA isolated from serum, it appears that the secretory molecule contains all of the antigenic determinants present on the α chains of serum IgA, and vice versa. However, when these two molecules are compared using antisera made against SIgA, significant differences are observed. By gel diffusion analysis, the secretory molecule shows a unilateral spur over serum IgA as illustrated in Fig. 4-1. This pattern, called a reaction of partial immunological identity, indicates that the secretory molecule contains an extra antigenic determinant which is not present on serum IgA. Such anti-SIgA antisera can be rendered specific for the extra determinant [secretory component (SC)] by absorption with serum IgA or whole normal human sera. Care must be taken in absorbing with whole normal sera and myeloma IgA because frequently small amounts of SIgA are present and may absorb out all of the anti-SC antibodies. The extra antigenic determinant present on the intact SIgA is immunologically identical to that present on the SC molecule which is found free in the secretions of newborns or patients with agammaglobulinemia.

In the human, approximately 85% of the IgA molecules in colostrum contain SC. In addition to the major 11S IgA, secretions contain higher polymers (15–18S) of IgA which also have SC determinants, but most of the 7S IgA does not. As already mentioned, no evidence has been found for SC on IgG and IgE, but a significant fraction of IgM present in the secretions does contain bound SC. Immunological studies in several other species including the monkey, rabbit, dog, cow, guinea pig, and mouse have also demonstrated an extra antigenic determinant on IgA from secretions, which is probably analogous to the human SC, although this has not been established with certainty in all cases (see also Chapter 3).

38

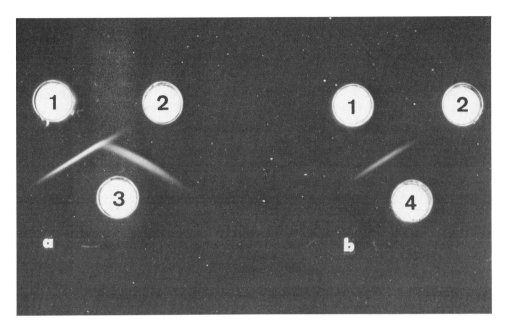

Fig. 4-1. Ouchterlony gel diffusion experiment showing immunological relationship of secretory and serum IgA. (a) Well 1: isolated secretory IgA; well 2: serum IgA; well 3: antisecretory IgA. (b) Well 1: isolated secretory IgA; well 2: serum IgA; well 4: antisecretory IgA absorbed with myeloma IgA.

In addition to SC which is unique to the 11S molecule in external fluids, SIgA also shares with serum IgA polymers so-called polymer specificity. Thus, certain rare antisera contain polymer-specific antibodies and demonstrate a spur of the SIgA and polymer serum IgA over isolated 7S IgA. With at least one such antiserum this reactivity was shown not to be due to antibodies to J chain (see Chapter 3) which is common to SIgA and polymer serum IgA.

At least four separate antigenic determinants associated with human SC have been described by P. Brandtzaeg during the course of extensive studies of the antigenic properties of SIgA and SC. Antisera made against free secretory component (FSC) may contain antibodies which show specificity for an antigenic determinant accessible in the FSC but inaccessible when SC is covalently linked in the native SIgA molecule. This is the so-called I (for inaccessible) antigenic determinant. The I determinant can be detected following treatment of SIgA with agents, such as acid or low concentrations of urea, which results in sufficient uncoiling of the native molecule to reveal an otherwise buried determinant. The I determinant can also be exposed by mild reducing conditions which do not dissociate a significant amount of the SC. However, at higher concentrations of reducing agents, for example above 0.15 M β-mercaptoethanol (βME), this determinant is destroyed. The I determinant is of some practical importance since I-specific antisera can be used to quantitate FSC in biological fluids even in the presence of SIgA (see also Chapter 3).

Covalently bound SC and FSC share two antigenic determinants referred to as A1 and A2. These can be distinguished from one another by their susceptibility to disulfide reduction; the A1 determinant is destroyed at about 0.15 M βME, while the A2 determinant is highly resistant to reduction. An additional rare determinant has been termed C (for conformational). This appears to be specific for SC covalently bound in the SIgA molecule.

As was mentioned earlier, antisera made against either FSC or 11S SIgA not infrequently contains antibodies to contaminants even though the immunizing preparations were apparently homogeneous as tested by various physical and immunological techniques. It appears, as is so often the case, that the rabbit is more adept at detecting impurities than the investigator. Particularly common "contaminants" are antibodies against blood group substances, lactoferrin, and a poorly characterized component referred to as macromolecular component (MMC). In order to use antisera containing these contaminating antibodies to localize or quantitate SC, it is necessary to first absorb with purified preparations of the contaminating substances. A description of the methods available for obtaining the preparations used for absorption is beyond the scope of this monograph, and the reader is referred to the review by the author which is listed in the references at the end of this chapter.

REFERENCES

Brandtzaeg, P.: "Human Secretory Immunoglobulins. III. Immunochemical and Physicochemical Studies of Secretory IgA and Free Secretory Piece," *Acta Path. Microbiol. Scand.,* 79B:165, 1971.

Brandtzaeg, P.: "Local Formation and Transport of Immunoglobulins Related to the Oral Cavity," in *Host Resistance to Commensal Bacteria,* ed. by T. MacPhee, Churchill Livingstone, Edinburgh, 1972.

Tomasi, T. B., and J. Bienenstock: "Secretory Immunoglobulins," *Advances in Immunology,* ed. by F. J. Dixon and H. G. Kunkel, Academic Press, New York, 1968, Vol. 9, p. 1.

Chapter 5

The Development

of the Secretory System

THE ORIGIN OF ANTIBODIES IN THE NEWBORN

Among mammals there is considerable variation in the type, amount, and route by which the various immunoglobulins are transferred from mother to fetus in utero. Some species' differences are illustrated in Table 5-1. Transport is selective in most species and occurs either via the placenta

Table 5-1

The relative amounts and durations of transmission of antibodies in the pre- and postnatal periods in different species [a]

Species	Amount and route of prenatal transmission	Amounts and durations of post-natal transmission
Horse, goat, sheep	0	+++ (24 hrs)
Pig	0	+++ (24–36 hrs)
Wallaby	0	+++ (180 days)
Dog, cat	+ (unknown)	++ (1–2 days)
Mouse	+ (yolk sac)	++ (16 days)
Rat	+ (yolk sac)	++ (20 days)
Fowl	++ (yolk sac)	++ (<5 days)
Guinea pig	+++ (yolk sac)	0
Rabbit	+++ (yolk sac)	0
Man, monkey	+++ (placenta)	0

[a] Modified from F. W. R. Brambell, in *The Transmission of Passive Immunity from Mother to Young*, American Elsevier Publishing, Co., Inc., New York, 1970, p. 14.

as in the human and monkey, or yolk sac as in the mouse, rat, and rabbit. The permeability of the placenta has been correlated, although not perfectly, with its anatomic structure, i.e., the number of anatomical layers separating the maternal and fetal circulations. For example, in species such as the cow, sheep, goat, and pig, five or six layers separate the maternal

41

and fetal circulations. The placentas of these species are essentially impermeable to any type of immunoglobulin and their newborn are, therefore, agammaglobulinemic. These species receive maternal antibodies only after birth via the colostrum since their gastrointestinal tracts remain permeable to immunoglobulins for 1–2 days following parturition. The importance of maternally derived (colostral) antibody is evident from the observations of Theobald Smith in early 1920 that nearly 75% of newborn calves die of E. coli sepsis within a few days of birth if prevented from suckling. The placenta and yolk sac of other species are selective and only certain classes of immunoglobulins reach the fetus. In the human, the placenta is two cell layers thick and only maternal IgG passes into the fetal circulation. Good evidence is now available that this selective transport results from specific receptors present on the Fc portion of the IgG molecule which are not present on the other immunoglobulin classes. Even among IgG subclasses there are differences in permeability, IgG_2 molecules being deficient in their ability to pass the human placenta compared with the other subclasses (see also Table 3-1, Chapter 3). In man, very little absorption of immunoglobulins occurs postpartum. Other animals such as the mouse and rat receive maternal antibodies both via the placenta in utero and postpartum from colostrum and milk.

In most mammals the serum of the unsuckled newborn is severely deficient in IgA. It appears that of the three major immunoglobulins (IgG, IgA, and IgM), the placenta of most species is more impermeable to IgA than to the other immunoglobulins. The umbilical cord blood of the normal full-term human newborn has an IgG level which approaches or slightly exceeds that in the maternal circulation; IgM is about $\frac{1}{20}$th and IgA is less than $\frac{1}{100}$th of the normal adult serum levels. IgD and IgE are not detectable in newborn serum by most currently available methods. By special methods such as the double-antibody immunoassay, it has been possible to detect small amounts of IgE in cord sera (35–40 nanograms per milliliter). When IgA is easily detected in cord serum (i.e., by gel diffusion analysis) usually there is either a placental leak allowing maternal blood to enter the fetal circulation or an intrauterine infection resulting in the synthesis of IgA by the fetus. In fact, increased cord blood levels of both IgM and IgA have recently been used clinically as an indication of an infection in the newborn acquired in utero. For example, the cord blood of infants born with rubella or cytomegalic virus infection frequently have high levels of IgM and IgA.

In vitro organ culture of tissues from human fetuses obtained at various gestational ages has shown that the first immunoglobulin synthesized is IgM. Synthesis of IgM begins at about 10 weeks, while IgG is first detectable at 12 weeks. In the normal fetus, no evidence of IgA synthesis occurs in cultures up to 32 weeks. Using the fluorescent-antibody technique, a virtual absence of IgA-containing cells has been noted in peripheral lymphoid tissues (spleen and lymph nodes) and also in secretory organs such as the gut and respiratory tract. Similar fluorescent findings have also been reported for mice and cows. Thus, it appears that the fetus and newborns of most species are more agammaglobulinemic with respect to IgA than to the other major immunoglobulins. However, a small amount of synthesis of IgA may occur in the human fetus as evidenced by studies on amniotic fluid. Using a genetic factor, Am2(+), which is inherited as a co-dominant marker on the α2 chain (see Chapter 3 for discussion of genetic markers on IgA, it has been demonstrated that, in selected families, the Am2(+) factor is present in the amniotic fluid and not the maternal serum. Thus the gene for Am2(+) must have been inherited from the father and the IgA synthesized by the fetus.

In contrast to mature plasma cells which contain cytoplasmic immunoglobulins, B lymphocytes bearing surface immunoglobulins are present in early fetal life. For example, in the human, B cells with surface IgM can be identified by 9.5 weeks of fetal age, and by 14.5 weeks the numbers of IgM, IgG, and IgA positive cells in hematopoietic tissues are essentially the same as in the adult. It seems likely, therefore, that B lymphocyte development is a normal maturation phenomenon which is independent of antigenic stimulation. In this regard, B cell development is similar to that of the T cell which first appears in the thymus at about the same time in fetal life as B cells are first detected (9–10 weeks). In the chicken, B cells having surface IgM are first seen in the bursa of Fabricius about 14 days of incubation (7 days before hatching). They develop from stem cells that have migrated to the bursa from the yolk sac. Thus, in the chicken, the bursa is a *central* lymphoid tissue analogous to the thymus gland. The mammalian homologue of the avian bursa has not been definitely identified, but the gut-associated lymphoid tissues and the bone marrow have both been suggested as possibilities.

Simply stated, the current hypothesis covering the development of the immunoglobulin system is as follows. Stem cells of hematopoietic origin (yolk sac, bone marrow) migrate to the central lymphoid tissues early in fetal life (around the ninth week in the human) and there differentiate into T cells (in the thymus) and B cells (in the bursa). Differentiation of T and B cells is dependent on the microenvironment of the central lymphoid organ and may involve the elaboration of an epithelial cell hormone. Once maturation has reached a certain stage, the central lymphoid cells populate peripheral tissues as depicted in Fig. 5-1. It is thus the central organs that supply the remainder of the body with immunocompetent T and B lymphocytes. The B lymphocytes are most easily recognized by the presence of surface immunoglobulins. They do not undergo expansion and development into plasma cells until directly stimulated by antigen. Presumably a

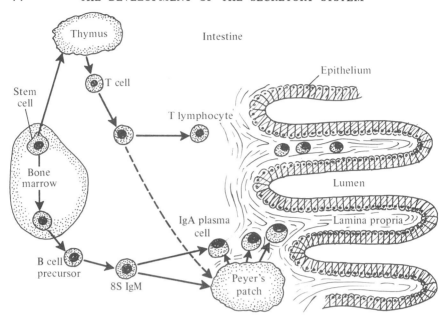

Fig. 5-1. Schematic representation of the possible sites of origin of cells in a secretory organ such as the intestine. 8S IgM refers to the immunoglobulin on the surface of the earliest B cell precursor which subsequently differentiates into a B cell with IgA on its surface. On antigenic contact the IgA B cells then differentiate into an IgA-secreting plasma cell.

lack of antigenic challenge is the reason for the paucity of plasma cells in the fetus and newborn of most species. It seems likely that the surface immunoglobulins on B cells represent receptors for antigen and that the eventual antibody formed by a cell is similar or identical to its surface receptor. The T cells lack easily detectable immunoglobulins, and the nature of their antigen receptors has not been elucidated. However, they do possess other identifiable surface components, such as the theta antigen. The concept of central lymphoid tissues and the early development of immunocompetent T and B cells in the absence of antigenic stimulation is fundamental to the clonal selection theory of antibody formation.

The concentration of IgA in human secretions increases with age more rapidly than the concentration of IgA in serum. Serum IgA levels are about 25% of adult values by 6 months of age, 50% by the end of 4 years, and they reach normal adult levels by 5–15 years (see Fig. 5-2). IgA can be detected in secretions such as tears and saliva by gel diffusion analysis as early as 8–10 days after birth at a time when serum IgA appears to be absent by this technique. In one study, 92% of normal infants had adult levels of IgA in their saliva by 1 month of age, although other studies suggest a somewhat more prolonged maturation of the

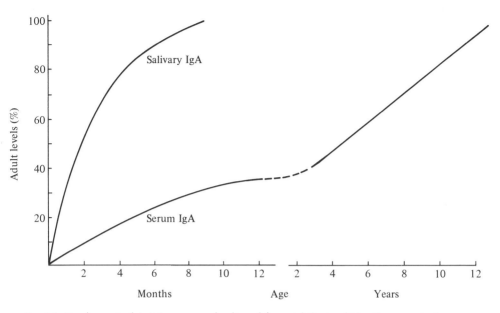

Fig. 5-2. Development of IgA in serum and saliva of human following birth. The concentration of IgA in the saliva reaches adult levels more rapidly than that in the serum.

secretory system. The more rapid development of IgA in secretions than in serum could be related to the greater antigenic stimulation which occurs initially at the mucous membrane. In this regard, a striking example of the effect of the degree of antigenic challenge on the secretory system is seen in studies on the development of the gut lamina propria cells in germ-free mice. In conventionally fed mice, the intestinal lamina propria and mesenteric lymph nodes begin to develop plasma cells containing IgA around 15–25 days after birth. Following the initial appearance of IgA cells in the GI tract, there is a very rapid proliferation of cells over the next 3–4 weeks, and by about 40 days of age, the numbers of lamina propria plasma cells closely approximates that found in the adult. Fluorescent-antibody studies on the mouse GI tract during development are illustrated in Fig. 5-3. On the other hand, animals maintained in a germ-free environment and therefore subjected to diminished antigenic stimulation have a markedly delayed appearance of IgA plasma cells in the intestinal mucosa. At 2 months of age, the number of plasma cells are about 10% of the age-matched conventionally fed controls.

Secretory component synthesis can be demonstrated in the human by the 7th week of fetal life. This is well before any immunoglobulin synthesis occurs by the fetus and even before transport of immunoglobulins from the mother, which begins at about 8 weeks. Figure 5-4 shows a photograph

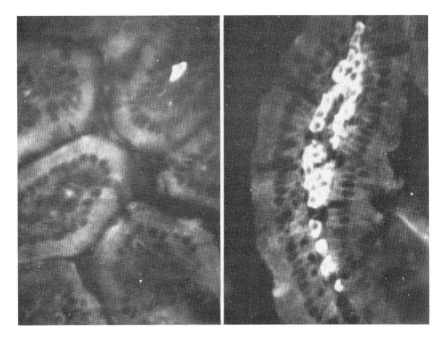

Fig. 5-3. (a) Tranverse section of several intestinal villi from a 15-day-old mouse. Many villi were scanned and only one IgA plasma cell was found. (b) Longitudinal section of a villus from an adult mouse illustrating the large number of IgA plasma cells present in the intestinal mucosa of conventional animals. Fluorescent photomicrographs. ×250. (Data from C. A. Mattioli and T. B. Tomasi, *J. Exp. Med.*, 138:452, 1973).

of a 16-week-old fetal kidney which was stained with a fluorescent anti-secretory component antiserum. This fetus, obtained by therapeutic abortion, showed no evidence of IgA cells in any organ. The presence of SC in fetal tissues and its occurrence in newborn saliva in the absence of detectable immunoglobulins indicates that synthesis of SC does not require stimulation by IgA or other immunoglobulins. Moreover, these observations vividly illustrate that the cell of origin of SC is not the lymphoid-plasma cell.

SOURCES OF ANTIGENIC STIMULATION

From the preceding discussion, it is obvious that antigenic stimulation is an important determinant of the immune response. In fact, it seems likely that it is mandatory for normal serum and secretory antibody formation. In the upper respiratory and gastrointestinal tracts, inhaled or ingested antigens can traverse the mucosa by an as yet undefined mechanism and directly stimulate the lamina propria lymphoid cells which are just below

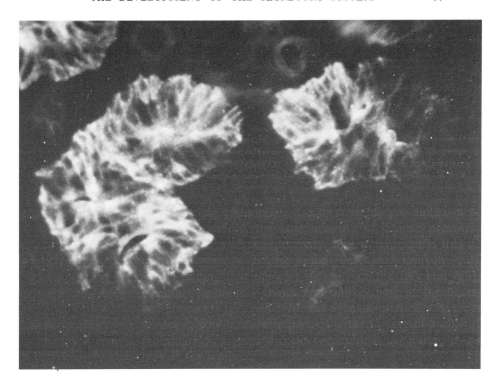

Fig. 5-4. Kidney from a 16-week-old human fetus stained with a fluorescein labelled antisecretory component antiserum.

the basement membrane of the epithelium. Evidence for this has been obtained for some nonviable antigens which, when locally deposited on the mucous membrane, elicit the production of antibodies in secretions and not in serum. In the more usual case, for example, with killed influenza virus, deposition on the respiratory mucosa leads to SIgA antibodies in secretions, and serum antibodies are also formed, primarily of the IgG and IgM types. It is also possible that certain antigens may be absorbed and stimulate antigen reactive cells in the Peyer's patches and/or mesenteric nodes. These cells could then migrate via the circulation to the GI tract and produce secretory antibody. (See below for a discussion of role of Peyer's patches and mesenteric node cells.)

Many antigens, when administered parenterally, are able to reach, via the circulation, secretory sites and elicit the local production of SIgA antibodies. The chemical properties of an antigen which determine whether or not it will stimulate secretory antibodies when administered parenterally have not been carefully investigated. However, it is known that the dosage of the antigen administered is of considerable importance. For example, with parenterally administered influenza virus vaccine, the secretory anti-body response is dose-related; the usual amount used in systemic immunization produces little or no nasopharyngeal antibody, whereas doubling the dose regularly elicits SIgA anti-influenza antibody in nasal fluids.

There is now extensive experimental evidence which indicates that both the respiratory and the digestive tracts of many animals allow penetrations of small but biologically significant amounts of antigenically active macromolecules. A good example is data recently obtained on the absorption of the enzyme, horseradish peroxidase (molecular weight 40,000), by the rat small intestine. It has been known for some time that, as a mechanism of acquiring passive immunity, the small intestine of the neonatal rat absorbs large quantities of immunoglobulins for about three weeks. Allegedly, absorption then ceases because the mucous membrane of the intestine matures and becomes a nearly complete barrier to the passage of macromolecules. However, that this is not the case with some proteins (e.g., horseradish peroxidase) was shown using everted gut sacs to compare the transport of the enzyme in adult and neonatal animals. Absorption in the adult jejunum and ileum actually exceeded that in the corresponding segments from neonatal animals, and electron microscopic studies showed that absorption in the adult intestine was by endocytosis similar to that in neonatal animals. Other examples of a less quantitative nature can be cited in which biologically active molecules such as insulin are absorbed as evidenced by a systemic response (i.e., hypoglycemia). Thus, following the oral administration of antigens, the antibody response may be of two types. One type is the *parenteral* response in which serum antibodies, usually IgM followed by IgG, are produced in the spleen and peripheral lymph nodes as a result of the absorption of antigenically intact macromolecules. The second or *enteric* type of response results from direct antigenic stimulation of lymphoid tissues in the gut lamina propria. Antibodies formed in the enteric response may then diffuse or be transported in two directions, either into the lumen as SIgA antibody or into the serum as serum IgA antibody. The evidence for this two-way transport of antibody will be discussed in Chapter 6. A mixed type of response also occurs in which there is both parenteral and enteric antibody synthesis. This is probably the most common type of response.

ORIGINS OF LYMPHOID-PLASMA CELLS IN THE SECRETORY SYSTEM

Gowans and Knight first demonstrated in 1964 that there were two species of lymphocytes in the thoracic duct lymph of rats. By labelling cells with tritium and injecting them intravenously, they showed that the small lymphocytes homed to peripheral lymphoid tissues such as lymph node and spleen, whereas the larger, immature, blast-like lymphocytes (> 8 mμ in diameter) migrated primarily to the lamina propria of the gut. More recent work has shown that within about two days after caudal immunization (hind foot pads, gluteus, flanks) and before significant serum antibody can be detected, the thoracic duct contains large numbers (10–15%) of the lymphoid blast-like cells (immunoblasts). The origin of these cells is not certain, but it is possible that they are derived from Peyer's patches and/or mesenteric nodes (see below). These cells can be labelled by short-term culture in vitro in the presence of radioactive precursors of DNA such as H^3-thymidine or I^{125} iododeoxyuridine. When labelled cells are injected intravenously into syngeneic recipients, they home predominantly to the small bowel as determined by autoradiography and scintillation counting of organs. By this technique it can be determined that four or five immunoblasts homed to the small bowel for every one that reached peripheral lymphoid tissues. Presumably, these lymphocytes give rise to IgA-type plasma cells although, unfortunately, this was not directly demonstrated in these studies.

Transfer of lymphoid cells obtained from Peyer's patches from rabbits of one allotype into lethally irradiated recipients of another allotype has shown that the large immature Peyer's patch lymphocytes which do not contain cytoplasmic immunoglobulins migrate to the GI tract and give rise to IgA cells. In these studies the allotype was used as a marker for donor cells just as the radiolabel was employed in the previously quoted studies. Some of the injected cells are also found in the spleen and here they also differentiate into IgA cells. Only cells from the Peyer's patches give rise to IgA cells; an equal cell inocula derived from peripheral blood or lymph nodes seeded the spleen where they differentiated into IgG cells. Some illustrative data are summarized in Table 5-2. Similar studies utilizing mesenteric lymph node cells also show that these cells behave in their homing properties like Peyer's patch cells. Thus, it appears that Peyer's

Table 5-2

Equal cell inocula of rabbit lymphocytes from Peyer's patches and popliteal lymph node cells injected into irradiated rabbits of a different allotype. Plasma cell counts made on spleen and gut by immunofluorescence. Donor cells recognized by allotypic markers employing a fluorescent antiallotype antiserum.[a]

Source of cells	Spleen, % of donor cells containing		Gut Lamina propria	
	IgG	IgA	IgG	IgA
Popliteal lymph nodes	74	8	few	0
Peyer's patch	13	77	few	many

[a] Data from S. Craig and J. Cebra, J. Exp. Med., 134: 188, 1971.

patches and mesenteric node lymphoblasts are already committed to the synthesis of IgA and, moreover, they either have a greater affinity for gut tissues or an enhanced ability to proliferate there compared with other lymphoid cells. It has been essentially excluded that specific antigen present in the GI tract is the sole determining factor in cell localization since immunoblasts home to the lamina propria of unsuckled neonatal animals removed by Caesarian section and to subcutaneous abdominal implants of syngeneic fetal gut. In both models the gut is sterile and presumably antigen-free. However, this does not exclude a role for antigen in determining cell migration patterns under physiological conditions. The ability of immunoblasts to localize in isolated segments of bowel indicates that the transmittance of those cells is an inherent property of the small gut, perhaps dependent on complementary receptors on the immunoblasts and vascular endothelium of the intestine. Some of these relationships are depicted in Fig. 5-1.

Current theories of antibody formation suggest that the early B cell precursor lymphocytes which arise from stem cells in the bone marrow have IgM on their cell surface, probably low molecular weight (8S) IgM. IgM-bearing lymphocytes subsequently differentiate into IgG and IgA precursor cells as shown in Fig. 5-5. It is not certain whether IgA cells

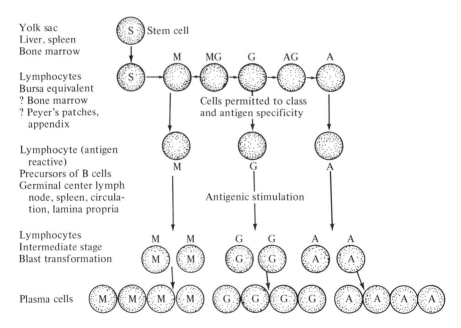

Fig. 5-5. Hypothetical scheme for the development of different classes of B cells and plasma cells. M = IgM, G = IgG, A = IgA. Symbol (A, G, or M) on outside of cell refers to surface immunoglobulins on B cells. Symbol on inside refers to plasma cell synthesizing the specific class of antibody.

originate directly from IgM cells or via an intermediate IgG stage as depicted in Fig. 5-5, or perhaps by both pathways. Experiments by Drs. Murgita and Mattioli in my laboratory, illustrated in Table 5-3 and Fig. 5-6, have shown that all IgA cells including those in the secretory system can be completely eliminated by treatment of mice from birth to early adulthood with anti-IgM antisera. This suggests that during development, a cell with surface IgM (and therefore eliminated by anti-IgM) preceded the IgA plasma cell. Administration of anti-IgA specifically suppresses only IgA synthesis in the spleen (see Fig. 5-7). Interestingly, the numbers of IgA cells in the gut lamina propria are only slightly depressed, probably because of a failure to reach high enough concentrations of the anti-IgA in the interstitial fluid of the GI mucosa.

Very little is known about the development of thymus-derived (T) lymphocytes in the secretory system. Since delayed type reactions occur locally in the respiratory and possibly gastrointestinal tracts in the absence of systemic cellular immunity (see Chapter 11), the effector T cells are

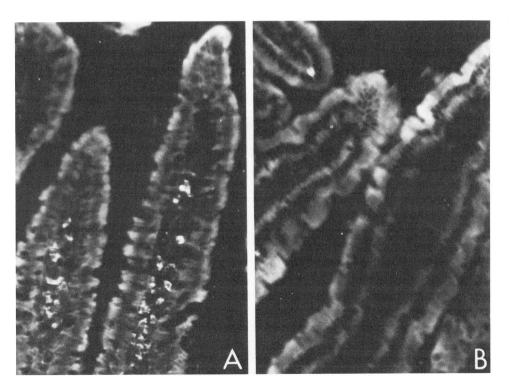

Fig. 5-6. Immunofluorescence of sections of intestine stained for IgA-containing cells. (a) Intestine from control mouse showing significant numbers of lamina propria IgA—plasma cells. (b) intestine from anti-IgM-treated mouse with lamina propria completely devoid of fluorescent cells. ×168. (Data from R. A. Murgita, C. A. Mattioli, and T. B. Tomasi, Jr., J. Exp. Med. 138:209, 1973.)

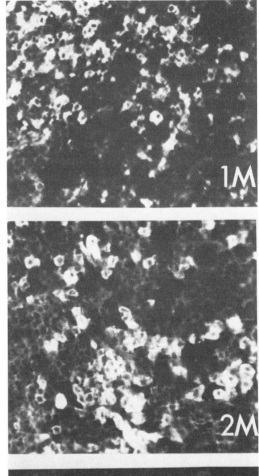

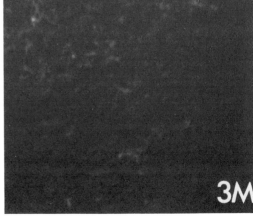

Fig. 5-7. Immunofluorescence of spleen sections from control, anti-IgA-treated, and anti-IgM-treated mice. Tissue sections were stained with rabbit anti-mouse IgM (M), IgA (A), and IgG (G). 1M, 1A, and 1G show spleen sections from mice treated with normal gammaglobulin. 2M, 2A, and 2G are spleen sections from anti-IgA-treated mice and demonstrate a selective absence of IgA-containing cells. Sections 3M, 3A, and 3G are from anti-IgM-treated mice and exhibit the virtual complete elimination of immunoglobulin-containing cells. ×175. (Data from R. A. Murgita, C. A. Mattioli, and T. B. Tomasi, Jr., *J. Exp. Med.*, 138: 209, 1973.)

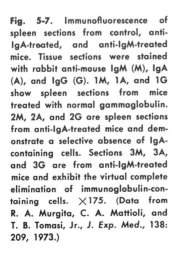

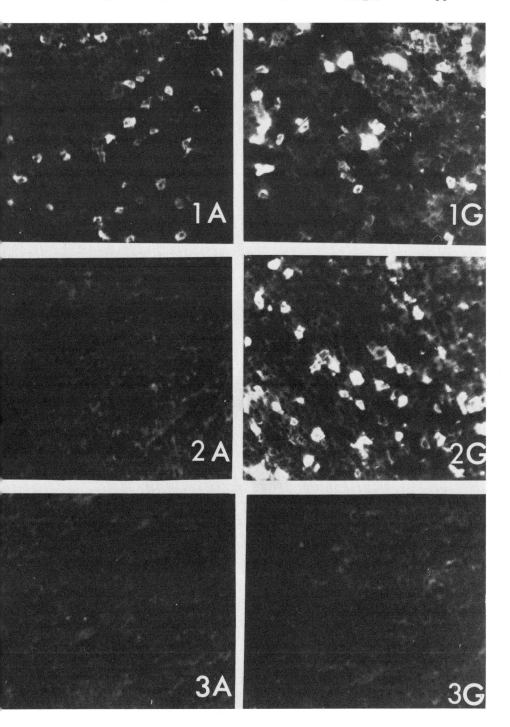

Table 5-3 [a]

Immunoglobulin class suppression in mice treated with anti-heavy-chain antisera.[b] Suppression of antibody formation by the administration of anti-immunoglobulin from birth to young adulthood. Anti-IgM suppresses antibody formation in all classes, whereas anti-IgA inhibits only the IgA response.

Treatment	Number of animals	PFC/10^6 spleen cells			Serum anti-SRBC antibody level [c]	Serum immunoglobulin level [d]				Intestinal lamina propria IgA cells/villus
		IgM	IgA	IgG		IgM	IgA	IgG$_1$	IgG$_2$	
Controls	19	77	78	101	3.6	7	4	110	11	10
Anti-IgA	15	50	0	60	3.3	3.3	0	60	16	8
Anti-IgM	13	13	0	0.5	0	0	0	30	3	8

[a] Data from R. A. Murgita, C. A. Mattioli, and T. B. Tomasi, Jr., J. Exp. Med. 138:209, 1973.

[b] Mice treated daily from birth to day 27 with 120 mg of globulin fraction from rabbit antisera or normal rabbit gammaglobulin (controls). Immunization with 5 × 10^8 SRBC on day 20. Plaque assay on day 30.

[c] Average reciprocal agglutination titer.

[d] Average highest reciprocal serum dilution giving precipitin band on Ouchterlony analysis.

presumably present on or near the mucous membrane in these organs. By a microneedle technique, thymidine ^{3}H can be injected subcapsularly into the frontal lobes of the neonatal mouse thymus, and the migration patterns of labelled thymic cells followed by radioautography. It has been found that in 1–2 day old mice about 74% of the cells in the mesenteric lymph node and 61% in Peyer's patches are of thymic origin, compared to 25% in the spleen. The greater thymic migration to the gut-associated lymphoid tissues has been tentatively attributed to the greater antigenic stimulation in the intestine during early life. In other studies employing fluoresceinated anti-θ antisera (θ is a marker for T cells in the mouse), over 90% of the Peyer's patch cells removed three days postpartum are T cells. It should be noted that these studies focused only on the mesenteric nodes and Peyer's patches and not the lamina propria, and they were restricted to the early neonatal period. It would be expected that, as B cells appear, the proportion of T lymphocytes would decrease considerably, and we have found that 70% of the Peyer's patch cells of the adult mouse are T cells. The experiments quoted above, demonstrating extensive migration of thymic lymphocytes to Peyer's patches, indicate that this organ, like other "secondary lymphoid" structures, is in large part dependent upon the thymus. This finding is contrary to the hypothesis that Peyer's patches are primary or central lymphoid tissues and strictly analogous to the bursa of Fabricius of birds. Much controversy centers around the site of the mammalial equivalent of the bursa, and the gut-associated lymphoid tissue (GALT) has been thought by several workers to be a likely candidate, although this is far from established. The reader interested in a more detailed discussion of this area should consult the recent review by M. D. Cooper and A. R. Lawton listed in the references at the end of this chapter.

REFERENCES

Cooper, M. D., and A. R. Lawton: "The Mammalian 'Bursa Equivalent'," in *Contemporary Topics in Immunobiology,* ed. by M. G. Hanna, Jr., Plenum Press, New York, 1972, p. 49.

Cooper, M. D., A. R. Lawton, and P. W. Kincade: "Developmental Approach to the Biological Basis for Antibody Diversity," in *Contemporary Topics in Immunobiology,* ed. by M. G. Hanna, Jr., Plenum Press, New York, 1972, p. 33.

Crabbe, P. A., H. Bazin, H. Eyssen, and J. F. Heremans: "The Normal Microbial Flora as a Major Stimulus for Proliferation of Plasma Cells Synthesizing IgA in the Gut," *Int. Arch. Allergy,* 34:362, 1968.

Craig, S. W., and J. J. Cebra: "Peyer's Patches: An Enriched Source of Precursors for IgA-Producing Immunocytes in the Rabbit," *J. Exp. Med.,* 134:188, 1971.

Gowans, J. L., and E. J. Knight: "The Route of Re-Circulation of Lymphocytes in the Rat," *Proc. Roy. Soc.,* 159:257, 1964

Hall, J. G., and M. E. Smith: "Homing of Lymph-Borne Immunoblasts to the Gut," *Nature,* 226:269, 1970.

Joel, D. D., M. W. Hess, and H. Collier: "Magnitude and Pattern of Thymic Lymphocyte Migration in Neonatal Mice," *J. Exp. Med.,* 135:907, 1972.

Mattioli, C. A., and T. B. Tomasi: "The Life Span of IgA Plasma Cells from the Mouse Intestine," *J. Exp. Med.* 38:452, 1973.

Moore, A. R., and J. B. Hall: "Evidence for a Primary Association Between Immunoblasts and Small Gut," *Nature,* 239:161, 1972.

Murgita, R. A., C. A. Mattioli, and T. B. Tomasi: "Production of a Runting Syndrome and Selective γA Deficiency in Mice by the Administration of Anti-Heavy Chain Antisera," *J. Exp. Med.,* 138:209, 1973.

Rogers Brambell, F. W.: in *The Transmission of Passive Immunity from Mother to Young,* North-Holland Publsihing Co. (American Elsevier Publishing Co.), New York, 1970.

Walker, W. A., K. J. Isselbacher, and K. J. Bloch: "Intestinal Uptake of Macromolecules: Effect of Oral Immunization," *Science,* 177:608, 1972.

Chapter 6

Metabolism of

Secretory Immunoglobulins

Origin of Secretory Immunoglobulins

The immunoglobulins present in external secretions may reach these fluids by one or both of two routes: local synthesis in lymphoid-plasma cells located in the interstitial tissues immediately adjacent to the mucous membrane and surrounding the glandular acini, or by transudation or active transport from serum. There is now good evidence that the majority of the IgA in secretions is synthesized locally. The concept of local synthesis of IgA is based on the following observations:

1. In certain cases, there is little or no correlation between immunoglobulin levels in serum versus external secretions. For example, during development following birth, levels of immunoglobulins in saliva and tears rise much more rapidly than those in serum, as was discussed in Chapter 5. In some situations, the IgA level of serum may be markedly elevated and yet the salivary concentration of IgA is normal or even low, e.g., some patients with disseminated lupus and IgA-type myelomas. As will be discussed in more detail in Chapter 9, there is often a dissociation between titers of specific antibodies in the serum and secretions. For example, it is possible by local mucous membrane application of killed viral antigens to produce SIgA antibodies in the absence of a detectable serum response.

2. In vivo studies in which I^{131}-labelled 7S serum IgA or 11S SIgA was injected intravenously into control subjects failed to demonstrate significant transport of IgA into salivary or nasal secretions. However, many external secretions contain small amounts of 7S IgA, and this is apparently transferred unaltered from serum. For example, in a metabolic study employing I^{131}-labelled 7S IgA, it was calculated that 96% of the total salivary IgA is synthesized locally, and that the small amount of 7S IgA which is normally found in saliva is derived from serum probably by "nonspecific" transudation through routes which are common to other serum proteins (see also Chapter 7—Transport of Immunoglobulins).

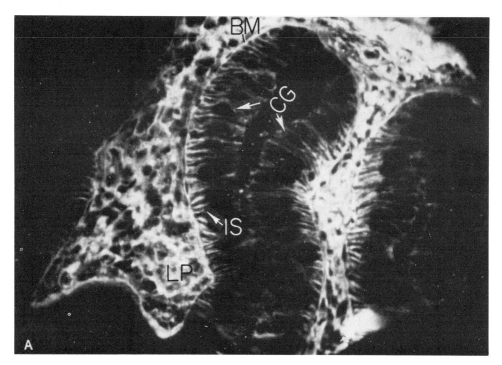

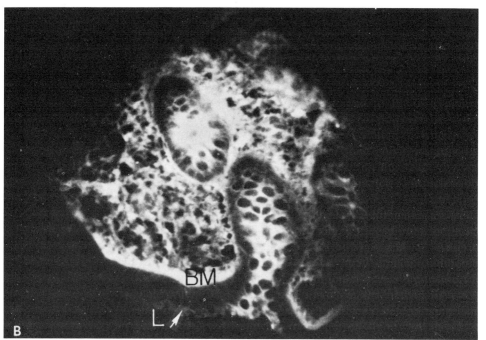

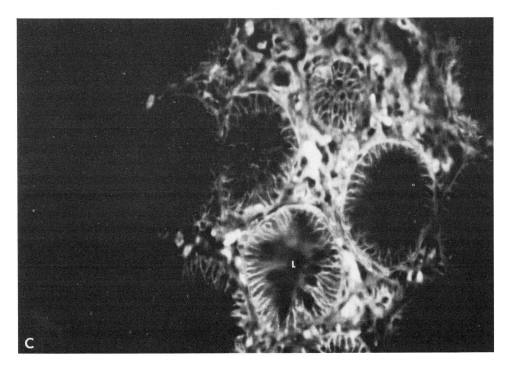

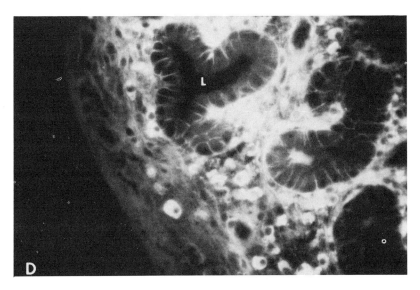

Fig. 6-1. Immunofluorescent localization of IgA in human colonic and nasal mucosa. (a, b, and c) Sections of colon. (d) Nasal mucosa stained with antiserum IgA. IgA fluorescence of plasma cells in lamina propria of colon and interstitial region of nasal mucosa. IgA is seen lying free in interstitial areas of both organs, along basement membrane (BM) and within the intercellular spaces (IS) between glandular epithelial cells. In (b), weak IgA fluorescence is seen along the luminal surface of the mucosa (L). In (c) and (d), the glands are cut in cross section with lumen (L) in center. Linear projections of IgA contained in intercellular spaces are clearly seen in these sections (Data from D. R. Tourville, R. H. Adler, J. Bienenstock, and T. B. Tomasi, Jr., *J. Exp. Med.*, 129:411, 1969)

Studies in which large amounts of normal human plasma are infused into patients who are agammaglobulinemic or newborn infants during exchange transfusions for erythroblastosis have yielded somewhat variable results. In general, these studies suggest that very little if any IgA (or other immunoglobulins) can be found in saliva following the plasma infusions. However, two of five patients with agammaglobulinemia showed small amounts of IgA in their salivas when their serum IgA was raised to high levels. IgG was not detected in the saliva of the two patients having IgA even though their serum concentration of IgG was artificially elevated to a greater extent than that of IgA. This suggests that transport mechanisms may exist which are relatively selective for IgA and probably also for IgM. Both IgA and IgM complex with SC which may act as a membrane receptor, facilitating the transport of these molecules. Support for this concept has also been obtained from fluorescent antibody studies, showing the presence of large amounts of both IgA and IgG in the interstitium surrounding the glandular acini in the respiratory or GI tract. However, only IgA is visualized in the intercellular spaces and lumen of the glands as shown in Fig. 6-1. In IgA-deficient patients, IgM is found in the same locations.

One interpretation of the above observations is as follows. IgA is selectively transported from the interstitial fluid of various secretory organs. As discussed later in this chapter and in Chapter 7, transport may be relatively specific for dimeric IgA, possibly because of the ability of the dimer to complex with SC. If this thesis is correct, then the concentration of IgA in secretions following an infusion will depend not only on the final serum concentration of IgA achieved, but also on the percentage of dimeric IgA in the preparation infused, as well as the permeability of the capillaries in the particular secretory tissues under study. Since it is known that local capillary permeability varies considerably from tissue to tissue, it would be expected that the amount of IgA transported into different secretions following infusion would vary. Unfortunately, experimental data on the permeability of monomer (7S) vs dimer (10S) IgA into various secretions are not presently available.

Another factor determining transfer of an infused protein into secretions can be termed *nonspecific transudation*. The mechanism by which this occurs and whether it is truly nonspecific is not clear. Usually it is visualized as occurring via holes or breaks in the capillary and/or mucous membrane epithelium. It is known that inflammation, including that induced by immune reactions involving complement, increases permeability both because of the release of relatively specific mediators such as histamine, as well as the morphological disruption of vessels and other elements which often accompanies invasion of tissues by inflammatory cells. In any case, this type of transudation is nonspecific in the sense that it is nonselective, and proteins of similar sizes such as 7S IgG and 7S IgA are excreted to approximately the same extent. Most capillaries are permeable to some extent to IgG, and large amounts of IgG (and other serum proteins) are seen lying free by fluorescent microscopy in most interstitial fluids. Since relatively small amounts of IgG are transported into secretions, these observations, along with the infusion studies mentioned above, support a selective and perhaps active transport of IgA.

3. In vitro organ culture techniques have been applied to secretory tissues derived from human and various animal species by a number of workers. In general, these studies employ radiolabelled amino acids which are added to small pieces of tissues maintained in vitro in an appropriate culture medium. After incubation the cells are disrupted and the incorporation of label into various immunoglobulins is then studied by immunoelectrophoresis followed by autoradiography as demonstrated in Fig. 6-2.

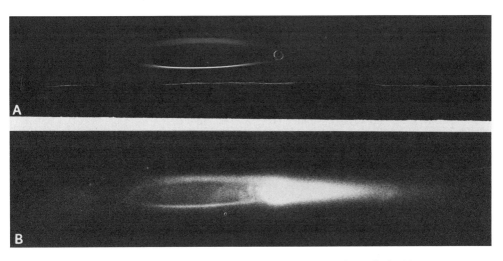

Fig. 6-2. Immunoelectrophoresis-radioautography of parotid tissue culture fluid. (a) immunoelectrophoresis of purified tissue culture fluid. Center well contains culture fluid to which isolated secretory 11S IgA has been added as a carrier. Upper trough contains antiserum against 11S IgA; lower trough contains antiserum against serum IgA. (b) Radioautograph of (a).

Synthesis (incorporation of label) into IgA and to a lesser extent IgG and IgM has been demonstrated in a variety of human tissues including those of the respiratory and GI tracts. Similar results have been obtained with GI tissues from various animals including the monkey, rabbit, mouse, goat, cow, pig, cat, and dog.

4. Loops of human intestine can be perfused ex vivo with oxygenated red cells in tissue culture media and C^{14}-labelled amino acids. Sections of gut, 6–8 inches in length, are obtained from grossly and histologically

normal tissue surrounding a localized carcinoma of the bowel. If perfusion is started in the operating room immediately after resection, the gut tissue will remain viable for periods of about 8 hours. Using this technique, it can be shown that synthesis occurs as determined by incorporation of C^{14} amino acids. Moreover, SIgA is secreted into the gut lumen while IgA without SC is added to the perfusion fluid, the latter being equivalent to the combined lymphatic-venous return. Pertinent to the discussion later in this chapter that intestinal IgA is synthesized as a dimer is the observation that about 70% of the IgA in the perfusion fluid is dimeric (10S IgA).

5. The relative concentrations of various plasma proteins in mesenteric lymph is proportional to their molecular size. An exception to this statement is IgA and to a lesser extent IgM which, as discussed later in this chapter (see also Fig. 6-5), is a result of local synthesis.

6. Fluorescent antibody studies have demonstrated an impressive predominance of IgA containing lymphoid-plasma cells in the interstitial regions of glands and the lamina propria of the mucous membranes (see Fig. 6-3). For example, in the human GI tract, there are approximately 20 IgA-producing cells per IgG cell, whereas in the peripheral lymphoid tissues (spleen and lymph nodes), IgG cells usually predominate about three to one (see Table 2-1 for cell counts in different tissues). An important finding is that various animal species including the rabbit, mouse, rat, guinea pig, cow, goat, sheep, pig, cat, dog, hamster, and hedgehog have all shown a similar predominance of IgA-type cells in the lamina propria of the GI tract. Thus the concept of a secretory system including its relationship to IgA is a general characteristic of many species.

The origin of the IgA in human and animal colostrum and milk has not been clearly established. It is known from organ culture experiments on monkey and rabbit mammary gland tissues that labelled amino acids are incorporated into IgA in vitro. Also, cells derived from human colostrum by low-speed centrifugation synthesize primarily IgA in culture. Experiments in rabbits have shown that the local injection of dinitrophenylated bovine gammaglobulin into mammary tissue elicits the production of DNP-specific milk antibodies of the IgA class. Foot pad immunization with the same antigen, on the other hand, fails to induce significant titers of colostral antibody. Both routes of injection result in serum antbodies primarily of the IgG and IgM class. Moreover, fluorescent antibody studies on mammary tissues from several species have demonstrated plasma cells containing IgA although they are not abundant. From all these data, there seems little doubt that local synthesis of IgA occurs in the mammary gland. However, the quantitative importance of local synthesis in supplying the large quantity of IgA which is normally found in the milk of many species has not been established. For example, in the first 6 months following parturition, roughly 0.5 grams of IgA are produced per day by the

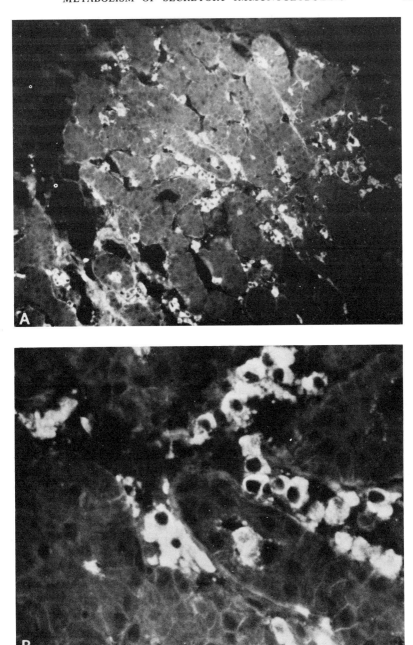

Fig. 6-3. IgA plasma cells in the interstitial region of lacrimal glands. (a) Low-power magnification, × 92. (b) High-power magnification, ×370. Similar accumulation of cells occurs in the submucosal and interstitial area between glandular acini in other secretory organs.

human lactating breast. A puzzling question, if local synthesis is subsequently shown to be quantitatively important, is the source of antigenic stimulation to the mammary lymphoid cells. One intriguing speculation is that cells in the gut, perhaps under the hormonal stimulus of late pregnancy, migrate to the mammary gland.

Another point which has not been completely settled is the proportion of the total IgA in gastrointestinal fluids which is derived from local synthesis. GI fluids contain, in addition to the predominant 11S IgA, significant quantities of 7S IgA, IgM, and IgG. There seems little question from the large numbers of IgA cells present in the lamina propria of the GI tract (20–30 IgA cells per IgG cell) that a significant proportion of the lumenal IgA is supplied by local synthesis. However, there is also evidence from studies in rats, dogs, and rabbits involving the passive transfer of immune serum that antibodies may reach the lumen of the GI tract from the circulation. The interstitial fluid surrounding the lamina propria cells is rich in IgG and this is apparently derived from serum. Thus, the intestinal capillaries are at least moderately permeable to 7S IgG and presumably 7S IgA. It is also known from studies on the intestinal lymph of dogs that significant amounts of IgG are found in this fluid which closely approximates the composition of interstitial fluid. Thus, an unknown proportion of the IgG and 7S IgA in intestinal secretions may well be derived by transudation from serum.

Secretory component is also synthesized locally but in a different cell type than IgA. The evidence that SC is synthesized by epithelial rather than plasma cells is as follows: (1) SC determinants can be visualized by fluorescent microscopy in epithelial cells of glandular acini and mucous membranes of secretory organs as shown in Fig. 6-4. The epithelial cells of the human salivary glands (acini and ducts), respiratory and GI tract mucosa, cervical and ovarian duct epithelial cells, biliary mucosa, kidney tubules, sweat glands, and thymus have all been shown to contain SC. Interstitial plasma-lymphoid cells do not contain SC. (2) SC is present in the secretions of newborns and agammaglobulinemic patients in the apparent absence of detectable immunoglobulins. (3) in vitro organ cultures of rabbit mammary tissue have demonstrated incorporation of C^{14} amino acids into SC obtained from the SIgA molecule. Kinetic studies in the same system have also suggested that IgA and SC are synthesized in different cell types.

There has been some dispute in the past as to whether the lamina propria plasma cells synthesize 7S IgA (monomer) which dimerizes subsequent to secretion from the cell, or whether dimerization occurs intracellularly. However, it now seems that the bulk of evidence points to the intracellular synthesis of a 10S IgA dimer. Several studies have shown that an individual colostral 11S SIgA molecule contains either k- or λ-type L chains, but not both. One would expect that, if plasma cells secreted 7S IgA which subsequently dimerized in the extracellular fluid, some mixed molecules would be formed as a result of the random association of monomers. Similarly, rabbit colostral IgA molecules obtained from animals which are heterozygous for L chain allotypes contain one allelic marker or the other, but not a mixture. Since mixed molecules can be produced by dissociation of a mixture of allotypes in guanidine and reassembly on subsequent removal of the guanidine, there is apparently no preferential association of molecules having the same allotype. Despite these observations, it is likely that some 7S monomer is secreted into the interstitial fluid by the lamina propria plasma cell but that it is not transported into secretions, perhaps because of its inability to complex with SC. Thus, in effect, monomer would be preferentially shunted via the lymphatics into the circulation. This possibility will be discussed in more detail later in this chapter.

In the human, both 7S and polymers of IgA coexist in normal sera as well as most IgA myeloma sera. It is not understood why some IgA molecules polymerize and others do not. One possibility is that some of the IgA molecules (7S monomers) have blocked SH groups, i.e., SH groups which are combined with other low molecular weight SH-containing compounds such as cysteine or glutathione. This type of SH blocking has been demonstrated with other proteins such as albumin, although no evidence for this could be obtained in one study of serum IgA. Another possibility is that J chain is required for dimerization and that the supply of this unique polypeptide chain is limited (see Chapter 3 for a discussion of J chain). Alternatively, two cell types may exist, one synthesizing J chain and polymeric IgA, the other monomer without J chain. Very recent studies employing isolated human SC labelled with a fluorochrome have demonstrated two types of cells in the human GI tract: one staining positively with SC, the other cell type failing to bind the labelled SC. The implication in these studies is that the positively staining cells contain dimer and J chain, and the negative cell, monomer IgA without J chain. However, as stated previously in Chapter 3, in the myeloma system where both monomer and polymer are the products of a single clone of cells, it seems unlikely that there would be two cell types differing in their ability to synthesize J chain.

Origin of IgG, IgM, and IgE in Secretions

In many secretions, IgG appears to be derived primarily from serum, but in others some is locally synthesized. For example, in normal parotid fluid, the small amount of IgG present appears to be derived entirely by transudation from serum. Similarly, in the normal GI tract the majority of IgG is probably derived by nonspecific transudation. This is suggested not only by the paucity of IgG-producing cells in the lamina propria, but

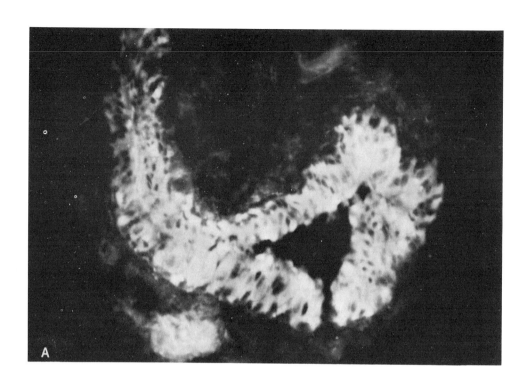

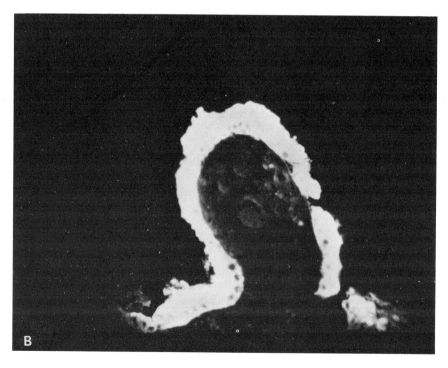

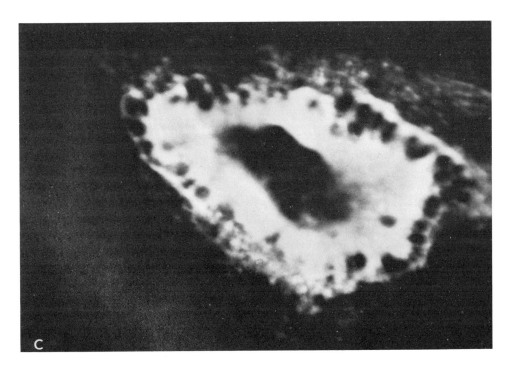

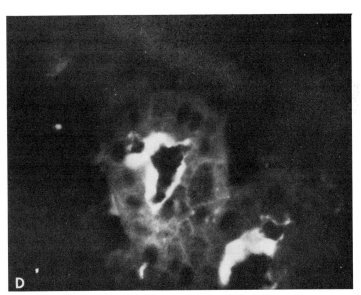

Fig. 6-4. Immunofluorescence localization of SC in various normal human tissues with fluorescein-labelled SC antiserum. (a) Section of parotid salivary gland tissue. Note SC staining localized in the epithelium of a ductule. (b) Section of gallbladder tissue showing intense SC staining in the epithelial cells. (c) Section of pancreas tissue showing SC staining in the ductular epithelial cells. (d) Section of lacrimal gland showing SC along the lacrimal border of the acinar epithelial cells.

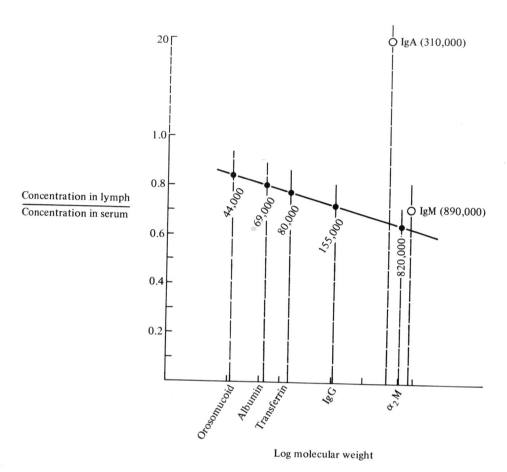

Fig. 6-5. Mesenteric lymph versus serum concentration ratios for different proteins as a function of their molecular weights. Molecular weight of proteins in parentheses. All of proteins except IgA and, to a lesser extent, IgM appear in lymph in concentrations inversely related to their molecular sizes. This indicates local production of IgA and IgM. (Modified from J. P. Vaerman and J. F. Heremans, *Immunology,* 18:27, 1970.)

also from studies of the intestinal lymph of dogs. In mesenteric lymph, the concentrations of IgG and other plasma proteins, except for IgA, are as expected if the formation of lymph is solely by a process of molecular sieving in which the different proteins occur in concentrations inversely related to their molecular size (see Fig. 6-5). These studies suggest that very little IgG is added to the intestinal lymph from synthesis by mucosal plasma cells. Also, in certain species such as the rat and rabbit, specific antibody infused intravenously does permeate into gastrointestinal secretions. With human nasal fluids, direct passage from serum has been demonstrated using I^{131}-labelled IgG. When inflammation of a mucous membrane occurs, such as following an upper respiratory tract infection or by simply rubbing the eye firmly several times, transudation of many serum proteins, including IgG, increases markedly. Thus, the degree of inflammation affects the passage of immunoglobulins from serum to secretions.

Another important factor determining the amount of a given immunoglobulin in a secretion is its susceptibility to enzymatic degradation. Although this is not a significant factor in parotid saliva, other fluids such as whole saliva and particularly gastrointestinal secretions possess significant proteolytic capacity. Experiments in mice involving the passive administration of antibody to Vibrio cholerae have demonstrated the rapid passage of both IgG and IgM antibodies into the gastrointestinal lumen in conventionally fed mice. In contrast, systemically administered antibodies cannot be detected in the intestinal contents of germ-free mice. On careful analysis, the absence of intestinal antibodies is not due to the impermeability of the germ-free intestine to the antibodies, but rather to the more rapid degradation of transmitted antibody. In studies in which IgG and IgM antibodies were injected into the lumen of isolated segments of mouse intestine and the segments returned to the peritoneal cavity for 1 hour of incubation, it was demonstrated that both IgG and especially IgM were rapidly degraded by germ-free small intestines and less so by the intestines from conventionally fed animals. Prior washing of the loops with saline to remove proteolytic enzymes resulted in nearly 100% recovery of added antibody. The reason for the reduced proteolytic activity in the intestine of conventional mice compared to germ-free animals has not been determined. The penetration of serum antibodies into the intestinal lumen and the proteolytic mechanism of immunoglobulin degradation have not been carefully studied in man.

In some tissues IgG is undoubtedly formed at least partly by local synthesis. This is shown by the presence of significant numbers of IgG-containing immunocytes and also by in vitro organ culture techniques which clearly demonstrate local synthesis. For example, gingival tissues surrounding the teeth normally contain large numbers of IgG cells (usually about 8 IgG per 1 IgA cell). It seems likely, therefore, that a significant part of the IgG found in gingival crevice fluid is derived from local production. The nasal mucosa immediately below the epithelium contains sizable numbers of IgG cells, while deeper, in mucosa surrounding the nasal glands, IgG cells are rare and IgA cells greatly predominate. IgG synthesis has also been demonstrated in the normal urinary tract. Following the induction of inflammation in the urinary bladders and kidneys of animals experimentally infected with E. coli, the amount of IgG synthesis increases markedly.

It seems likely that the majority of IgM present in most secretory fluids is synthesized locally. Fluorescent antibody studies in several tissues, including the salivary glands and GI tract, have shown a predominance of IgM compared with IgG cells. For example, in the human intestinal tract, IgM cells are approximately five times more numerous than IgG cells. Moreover, in diseases in which there is a selective deficiency of IgA, large numbers of IgM cells appear in the gut lamina propria and IgM seems to replace the IgA. Also, IgM is present in human parotid fluid in higher concentration than IgG. In view of the large size of IgM relative to IgG and the fact that at least 75% of IgM is intravascular (compared to 50% of the IgG), the higher concentrations of IgM in certain secretions such as saliva implies either selective transport from serum or, more likely, local synthesis.

Although the absolute concentration of IgE in saliva is very small, the ratio of the salivary to serum levels of IgE is high. Analysis of nasal fluids from individuals with allergies have also revealed high concentrations of IgE far in excess of what would be expected from simple transudation from serum. Immunofluorescent studies show larger numbers of IgE cells in secretory sites than in peripheral lymphoid tissues. For example, spleen and peripheral lymph nodes contain less than 1% IgE cells, whereas in the lamina propria of the gastrointestinal mucosa 3–5% of the total cells staining with an anti-L-chain antisera contain IgE. Thus, it appears that like IgA, IgE may also be synthesized predominantly in secretory sites. Local production of IgE and a high concentration in secretions (relative to that in serum) is perhaps not surprising in view of the reaginic function of the IgE molecule. It is likely that the interaction of an allergen, for example, ragweed pollen with its reaginic antibody fixed on the surface of tissue mast cells, initiates the release of pharmacologically active agents which are responsible for the symptoms of mucosal allergies such as hay fever.

SYNTHESIS OF SERUM IgA IN SECRETORY SITES

Important new information has become available suggesting that the intestinal lamina propria is a significant source of serum IgA in several species. Germ-free mice immunized orally with horse spleen ferritin develop large numbers of anti-ferritin-producing plasma cells, primarily of the IgA type, in the lamina propria of the gut. Very few antibody-containing cells are found in peripheral lymphoid tissues such as the spleen. Most important, the serum antibody response in these orally immunized animals is entirely in the IgA class. The same antigen given parenterally produces the usual sequence in the serum: IgM followed by IgG-type antibody, and in this case the cells producing these immunoglobulins, were found predominantly in peripheral lymphoid tissues such as the spleen, and only a few IgA producing antiferritin cells are seen in the GI tract. These experiments suggest that oral immunization stimulates IgA cells in the gastrointestinal tract that produce antibodies which are able to reach the serum probably by way of the intestinal lymphatics.

Good evidence that serum IgA originates in part in the GI tract has been obtained in irradiated mice. Marked decreases in serum IgA concentration, but not IgG or IgM, occur when mice are exposed to total body irradiation. The drop in serum IgA does not occur when the intestinal tract is shielded, and a significant decrease, selective for IgA, is observed when the bowel alone is irradiated. The decrease in IgA level is not due to leakage of serum IgA into the gut lumen, since the metabolic half-life of I^{131}-labelled IgA administered intravenously is normal. Moreover, although there is some decrease in the rate of synthesis of IgA by isolated segments of gut following irradiation, this is not of sufficient magnitude to account for the marked fall in serum IgA. By careful measurement of the lumenal content of IgA, it can be shown that irradiated mice continue to secrete approximately normal amounts of IgA into their intestinal tracts even though their serum IgA concentrations are severely depressed. By electron microscopy, widening of the intercellular spaces between epithelial cells is observed. The most likely explanation is that, following irradiation, abnormal communication develops between the interstitial spaces and the intestinal lumen, and IgA is preferentially shunted away from the serum and into the lumen, i.e., normally there is a two-way transport of locally synthesized IgA while in the irradiated animal the lumenal route is preferred.

Vaermans and Heremans have carefully quantitated the concentration of various serum proteins including immunoglobulins in the serum and intestinal lymph of dogs. As shown in Fig. 6-5, they found that all of the serum proteins measured appeared in mesenteric lymph in concentrations inversely related to their molecular size with the striking exception of IgA and to a lesser extent IgM. IgE and IgD were not measured in these experiments. It was concluded that, whereas most of the serum proteins found in mesenteric lymph were derived from serum by transudation across the intestinal capillaries, the major proportion (about 80%) of lymphatic IgA originated from local synthesis in the lamina propria lymphoid-plasma cells. From figures in the literature on the rate of secretion of intestinal lymph in the dog, it was calculated that the gut alone contributes approximately 138 mg/day of IgA to the plasma pool. This is approximately equal to the total intravascular pool of IgA. Thus, it appears that the intestinal tract of the dog is capable of supplying the majority of serum IgA. Similar results have been obtained in the guinea pig and rat. However, caution must be exercised in applying these findings to other species since there may be considerable differences in the contribution of the gut (and other secretory organs) to the serum IgA in various species.

One of the problems in ascribing a major role to the gut in producing serum IgA is that, in the human, approximately 85% of the serum IgA has a sedimentation coefficient of 7S. As mentioned above, the available evidence suggests that the majority of the IgA produced in secretory sites is secreted from the cells as a dimer. For this reason it is generally believed that peripheral lymphoid tissues (spleen, lymph nodes) are responsible for the synthesis of most of the circulating IgA. The bone marrow may also be important in IgA synthesis since, by rough calculations, as many as one-third of the IgA cells contributing to the serum pool may be located in the marrow. It is feasible that the GI tract and perhaps other secretory sites supply a large part of the 10–20% of polymeric IgA found in normal human sera. Another likely possibility in this author's view is that IgA is secreted from lamina propria cells in both monomer and dimer forms, but the 10S dimer is preferentially transported into the lumen, perhaps because of its ability to complex with SC, while the smaller and therefore more readily diffusible monomer is absorbed via the lymphatic into the serum (see Fig. 6-6). In this regard the author has found that the thoracic duct lymph-to-serum concentration ratio of IgA in the human is below one. This observation suggests that, unlike the dog and mouse GI tract, the human GI tract is not the major source of serum IgA. However, until more quantitative data for various proteins are available for human lymph, a significant contribution of the gut to the circulating pool of IgA cannot be

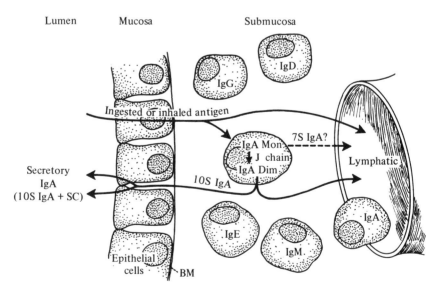

Fig. 6-6. Schematic drawing showing local synthesis and secretion of immunoglobulins at a secretory site such as the GI tract (see text for detailed description).

excluded. In other species such as the dog and cow, the serum IgA is predominantly dimeric and, accordingly, the conceptual problem discussed above is not encountered.

A final mechanism by which the secretory system could contribute to the serum IgA antibody response involves cell migration as depicted in Fig. 6-6. Following the oral administration of certain antigens in experimental animals, a higher percentage of the cells producing specific antibody in extra intestinal tissues such as the spleen are of the IgA type than when the same antigen is administered parenterally. Moreover, lymphoid cell migration in and out of intestinal tissues is now well established, as was discussed in Chapter 5. Thus, it seems likely that antibody-forming cells induced in the GI tract, which are primarily of the IgA type, may migrate to peripheral lymphoid tissues where they are a source of serum antibody.

REFERENCES

Bazin, H., P. Maldaque, E. Schonne, H. Bauldon, P. A. Crabbe, and J. F. Heremans: "The Metabolism of Different Immunoglobulin Classes in Irradiated Mice. V. Contribution of the Gut to Serum IgA in Normal and Irradiated Mice," *Immunology*, 20:571, 1971.

Brandtzaeg, P.: "Two Types of IgA Immunocytes in Man," *Nature New Biol.*, 243:142, 1973.

Bull, D. M., and T. B. Tomasi: "Deficiency of Immunoglobulin A in Intestinal Disease," *Gastroenterology*, 54:313, 1968.

Crabbe, P. A., and J. F. Heremans: "The Distribution of Immunoglobulin-Containing Cells Along the Human Gastrointestinal Tract," *Gastroenterology*, 51:305, 1966.

Crabbe, P. A., D. R. Nash, H. Bazin, H. Eyssen, and J. F. Heremans: "Antibodies of the IgA Type in Intestinal Plasma Cells of Germ-Free Mice After Oral or Parenteral Immunization with Ferritin," *J. Exp. Med.*, 130:723, 1969.

Franklin, R. M., K. R. Kenyon, and T. B. Tomasi: "Immunohistologic Studies of Human Lacrimal Gland: Localization of Immunoglobulins, Secretory Component and Lactoferrin," *J. Immunol.*, 110:984, 1974.

Genco, R. J., and M. A. Taubman: "Secretory γA Antibodies Induced by Local Immunization," *Nature*, 221:679, 1969.

Heremans, J. F., and P. A. Crabbe: "Immunohistochemical Studies on Exocrine IgA," in *Gammaglobulins. Structure and Control of Biosynthesis*, ed. by Killander, Almquist & Wiksell, Stockholm, 1967, p. 129.

South, M. A., M. D. Cooper, F. A. Wollheim, R. Hong, and R. A. Good: "The IgA System. I. Studies of the Transport and Immunochemistry of IgA in the Saliva," *J. Exp. Med.*, 123:615, 1966.

Tade, T., and K. Ishizaka: "Distribution of γE-Forming Cells in Lymphoid Tissues of the Human and Monkey," *J. Immunol.*, 104:377, 1970.

Vaerman, J. P., and J. F. Heremans: "Origin and Molecular Size of Immuno-globulin-A in the Mesenteric Lymph of the Dog," *Immunology*, 18:27, 1970.

Chapter 7

Transport of Immunoglobulins

A model for the route of transport of IgA across mucous membranes has been developed primarily on the basis of fluorescent antibody and electron microscopic studies. The fluorescent studies have utilized both antisera to α chains and SC, while the electron microscopic studies have employed a noninmmunoglobulin protein, horseradish peroxidase. Alpha chain determinants are found by fluorescent microscopy in the following locations: (1) Intracellularly in plasma cells in the interstitium of secretory glands and the lamina propria of the respiratory and gastrointestinal tracts (see Fig. 6-3). (2) In a linear pattern along the basement membrane of the mucosa, and lying free in the interstitial fluid (illustrated in Fig. 7-1). (3) Between epithelial cells in the intercellular spaces (see Fig. 6-1). (4) In the apical cytoplasm of the epithelial cells (see Fig. 6-1).

On the other hand, SC is visualized primarily in the cytoplasm of epithelial cells of secretory tissues, particularly concentrated in the area of the Golgi just above the cell nucleus. SC is also found on the surface "fuzz" layer which lines the mucous membrane of the respiratory and gastrointestinal systems as shown in Fig. 7-1. Although the distribution of IgA and SC, as noted above, has been obtained primarily from studies on the human GI tract, other tissues such as the nasal mucosa, salivary, and lacrimal glands show a similar distribution (see Figs. 6-1 and 6-4).

On the basis of these findings, it has been suggested that the IgA molecule follows the path outlined in Fig. 7-2. The dimeric IgA molecule traverses the basement membrane (BM) by diffusion. The BM probably represents a partial diffusion barrier since IgA accumulates along this structure. The IgA then passes through the intercellular space but is prevented from gaining direct access to the lumen by the epithelial tight junction. The tight junction is located at the apical limit of the intercellular space at which point the plasma membranes of two adjacent epithelial cells are in very close apposition. On electronmicrography, a typical tight junction is illustrated in Fig. 7-3. It has not been excluded, however, that a significant amount of IgA passes directly through the basal portion of epithelial cell cytoplasm. The fact that IgA is not visualized in the basal portions of the

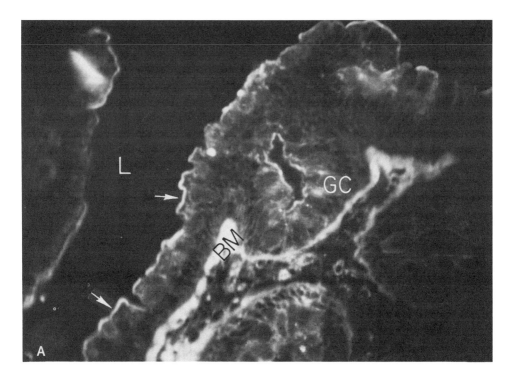

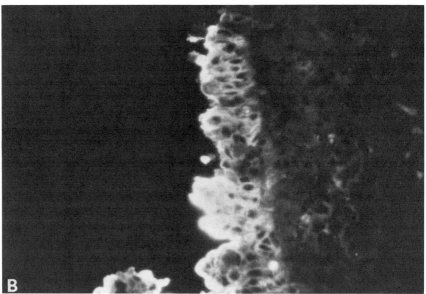

Fig. 7-1. Immunofluorescence localization of IgA and SC in human colonic and nasal mucosa. (a) Section of colon stained with dilute secretory 11S IgA antiserum. Linear SC staining on the surface of the epithelial cells (arrow) lining the lumen (L) and weak goblet cell (GC) staining is seen. IgA fluorescence is localized along the basement membrane area (BM). (b) SC staining on the surface of the nasal mucosa.

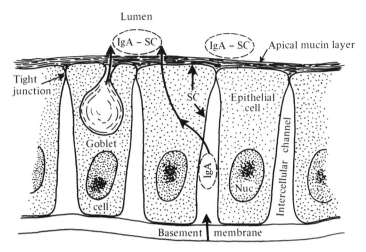

Fig. 7-2. A hypothetical model for the transport of IgA and SC across mucosal membrane epithelium.

epithelial cell may simply represent a concentration phenomenon. IgA concentrated in the narrow intercellular space may be clearly visible by fluorescent microscopy, whereas the same amount spread diffusely throughout the relatively large area at the base of the epithelial cell may not reach an antigen concentration sufficient to be visualized by the fluorescent technique.

An additional possibility especially applicable to the GI tract involves the release of immunoglobulins, particularly IgA, during the course of the normal shedding of epithelial cells. Mitosis of epithelial cells occurs predominantly at the base of the villus in the crypts of Lieberkühn, and the cells then migrate from the crypt to the tip of the villus. In the human it takes 2–4 days for an epithelial cell to reach the tip of the villus where it is dislodged into the lumen. Thus, the whole epithelial lining of the gastrointestinal tract is completely renewed every four days. During this process it would be expected that proteins (such as IgA) present in the intercellular spaces and within the epithelial cell itself would be released. It should be emphasized that the quantitative importance of this route or, for that matter, whether such a mechanism occurs at all has not been established. Moreover, there is no evidence that a similar maturation phenomenon occurs in other secretory organs such as the salivary glands which are capable of transporting sizable amounts of IgA.

The IgA present in the intercellular space diffuses or is transported from this space into the apical portion of the epithelial cell. This is consistent with the relatively heavy apical concentration of IgA seen by fluorescent microscopy. From the apex of the epithelial cell, the IgA transverses the luminal plasma membrane by a process that may involve reverse pinocytosis.

The passage of the enzyme horseradish peroxidase (M.W. 40,000) from the circulation through the mouse intestinal mucosa has been found to be similar to that described above for IgA. This enzyme has been utilized because of its ability to be reduced to an insoluble compound which can be visualized by both light and electron microscopy. In addition to the distribution mentioned above for IgA, horseradish peroxidase can also be visualized by electron microscopy enclosed in membrane-limited vesicular and vacuolar structures in the apical cytoplasm of epithelial cells. Studies involving this technique in the dogfish kidney have yielded similar findings to those described above for the GI tract, suggesting that this route may be a general one for the transport of proteins and perhaps other substances from serum to lumen. It is pertinent in this regard that small but significant amounts of horseradish peroxidase are absorbed into the circulation when introduced into the adult rat small intestine and the route appears to follow that outlined above. Thus, molecules in transport in both directions may follow a similar path.

Certain proteins such as horseradish peroxidase, even though they become concentrated in the apical cytoplasm of the gastrointestinal epithelial cell following intravenous administration, are apparently unable to reach the lumen, presumably because they are in large part digested in cytoplasmic vacuoles which are rich in hydrolytic enzymes (lysosomes). One speculative function for SC would be to protect the IgA molecule from intralysosomal proteolytic degradation, thus enabling it to take "the last step" into the lumen. As discussed in Chapter 3, in vitro experiments with various enzymes have shown that SIgA is more resistant to proteolysis than serum IgA. This concept would also be consistent with observations suggesting that one of the factors controlling the absorption of proteins from the adult gastrointestinal tract may be its susceptibility to proteolytic digestion within the phagolysosomal system of the intestinal epithelial cell.

SC is synthesized in the epithelial cell and reacts preferentially with dimeric IgA through covalent bonds. Just where in transport complexing of SC and lOS IgA occurs is not known. It could take place on the lateral

Fig. 7-3. Lacrimal gland: Survey electron micrograph of the human lacrimal gland demonstrating acinar epithelial cells (EP), with apical junctional complexes (arrowheads). In the interstium several plasma cells (PC) are seen ($\times 6015$). (L: acinar lumen); (SG: secretory granule); (*: interstitial space); (BM: basement membrane). Upper insert: Fluorescent micrograph ($\times 432$) of IgA-staining plasma cells (P) within interstitial area of lacrimal gland, IgA along basement membrane (*), in intercellular spaces (arrowheads) and within an acinar lumen (L). Lower insert: High magnification ($\times 73,080$) of an apical junctional complex consisting of a zonula occludens or tight junction (ZO) and a zonula adherens (ZA). (L: acinar lumen). (Data from R. M. Franklin, K. R. Kenyon, and T. B. Tomasi, Jr., J. Immunol., 110:984. 1973.)

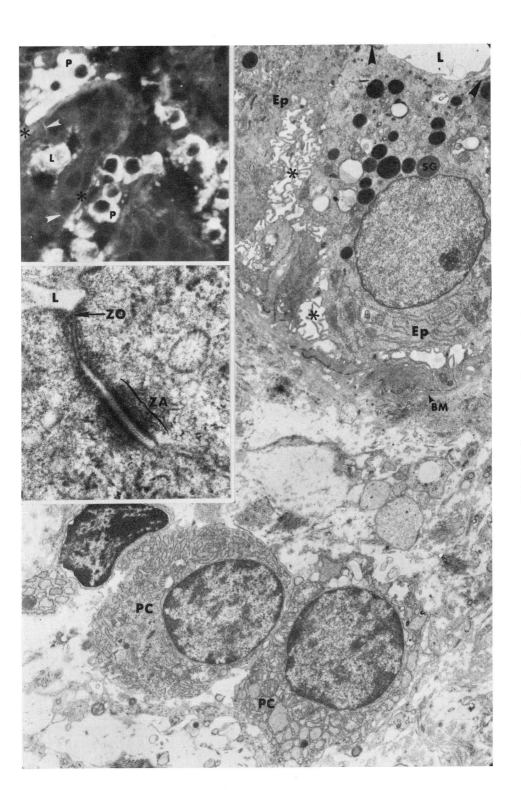

plasma membrane lining the intercellular space, and it is conceivable that SC localized on this membrane acts as a receptor for IgA.

IgM also appears to follow a route similar to IgA in its transport from interstitium to lumen. This can be most readily visualized in intestinal biopsies from IgA-deficient patients. These patients have nearly normal total numbers of lamina propria plasma cells, the majority of these cells containing IgM and μ chain determinants which are present in locations essentially identical to those described above for α chains.

Practically nothing is known about the route of transport of the other immunoglobulins (IgG, IgD, IgE). It may be that IgG, which is present in large amounts in the interstitial fluids of secretory organs, does not follow the IgA route, but rather small breaks occur in the mucosa which allows nonspecific leakage to occur. Some leakage may also occur during the process of epithelial shedding discussed before. Similar mechanisms may also be responsible for the presence in secretions of small amounts of serum proteins such as albumin which normally occurs in high concentrations in serum and interstitial fluids. A significant part of the 7S IgA present in certain external secretions such as saliva and nasal fluids may also follow the IgG route.

R E F E R E N C E S

Brandtzaeg, P.: "Mucosal and Glandular Distribution of Immunoglobulin Components: Differential Localization of Free and Bound Secretory Component in Secretory Epithelial Cells," *J. Immunol.*, 112:1553, 1974.

Farquhar, M. G., and G. E. Palade: "Junctional Complexes in Various Epithelia," *J. Cell. Biol.*, 17:375, 1963.

Poger, M. E., and M. E. Lamm: "Localization of Free and Bound Secretory Component in Human Intestinal Epithelial Cells. A Model for the Assembly of Secretory IgA," *J. Exp. Med.*, 139:629, 1974.

Reese, T. S., and M. J. Karnovsky: "Fine Structural Localization of a Blood-Brain Barrier to Exogenous Peroxidase," *J. Cell. Biol.*, 17:375, 1967.

Tourville, D. R., R. H. Adler, J. Bienenstock, and T. B. Tomasi: "The Human Secretory Immunoglobulin System: Immunohistological Localization of γA, Secretory, 'piece,' and Lactoferrin in Normal Human Tissues," *J. Exp. Med.*, 129:411, 1969.

Chapter 8

The Secretory System in Animals

Major difficulties are often encountered in defining IgA in various animal species. Most of the criteria that have been used in the past involve physicochemical or biological properties which are characteristic of human IgA: fast gamma electrophoretic mobility, high carbohydrate content, tendency to polymerize, failure to fix complement, and absence from cord sera. However, none of these criteria by themselves are sufficiently unique for characterization. For example, serum (and secretory) IgA in certain species such as the rat has a more rapid mobility than human IgA and there are other immunoglobulin classes such as IgE which do not fix complement or cross the placenta.

Of the characteristics mentioned above one of the most unique to IgA is the tendency to polymerize. The presence of intermediate (10–15S) polymers is typical of IgA and is not generally seen with the other immunoglobulins. However, complexes of low molecular weight rheumatoid factor (either IgG or IgM) with IgG have intermediate sedimentation properties and could easily be confused with IgA polymers, although this type of complex is relatively rare and has not yet been reported in animal sera.

Recently, several important new criteria have been established for characterizing an animal immunoglobulin as being analogous to that in the human. Perhaps the most absolute is amino acid sequence homology. At the present time this criterion is of limited usefulness with IgA because of the paucity of data available on the primary structure of the IgA molecule. Amino-terminal sequence data are not helpful in distinguishing between classes because of the variations in sequence normally encountered in this region even within a given immunoglobulin class. The C terminal sequence has been useful in identifying IgG, but with IgA difficulties are encountered because of the strong homologies between IgA and IgM in the C terminal region. Obviously, more extensive sequence studies will be necessary to characterize and distinguish IgA from IgM.

At the present time one of the best and most readily applied criterion is an immunological cross-reaction between human IgA and the suspected animal IgA using a specific antihuman IgA antiserum. Since the antigenic structure of a protein is ultimately closely related to its primary structure, this technique, in effect, provides an indirect method of determining amino acid sequence homologies. This criterion is a rather stringent one and, in general, if cross-reactivity is demonstrated, identification can be considered as definite. One drawback of this method is that in most cases cross-reactions are restricted to mammalian species, and the serum proteins of birds, reptiles, and fish do not in general give cross-reactions with the human proteins, although a few exceptions occur. For example, chicken IgM gives a good cross-reaction with human IgM.

Another useful, although not absolute, criterion is the predominance of the immunoglobulin in external secretions such as milk, tears, and saliva, although, as will be discussed below, IgA is not always the major immunoglobulin in secretions. For example, in bovine colostrum and milk, IgG is the predominant immunoglobulin. However, even in this species, IgA constitutes about 85% of the total immunoglobulin in saliva, nasal fluids, and lacrimal secretions. Moreover, in all species so far reported, the lamina propria of the gastrointestinal mucosa shows a vast predominance of IgA-containing cells.

A summary of the application of these various criteria to different species is shown in Table 8-1. The work of J. P. Vaerman in Belgium has greatly extended our knowledge of the IgA proteins in various species, and much of the data in this table is from his work. The interested reader is referred to an excellent review by Vaerman listed in the references at the end of this chapter.

ANIMAL SECRETORY SYSTEMS SIMILAR TO THE HUMAN

Several species have secretory systems quite analogous to that described in man (see Table 8-1). These include the monkey, rabbit, dog, guinea pig, rat, mouse, hamster, cat, and hedgehog. In these species IgA is the predominant immunoglobulin in secretions including colostrum and milk. The physicochemical properties of the major species of IgA in secretions are similar to those of human SIgA, i.e., it is intermediate in sedimentation (10–11S) and in the case of the monkey, dog, rabbit, and guinea pig, an additional polypeptide chain, probably analogous to SC in the human, has been described. Only with the monkey and the cow have immunological cross-reactions between human SC and the analogous animal protein been observed. However, the IgA of many species including the chicken, dolphin, and seal have been shown to complex with human SC.

It should be emphasized that the most frequent secretions studied in animals are colostrum and milk, and these are the very fluids which seem to show the most variations among species in regard to their relative content of the various classes of immunoglobulins. Other external secretions such as tears and saliva appear to be more uniform among the species in

Table 8-1

Summary of characteristics of IgA in different species[a]

	Polymer/monomer ratio in serum	Immunological cross-reaction with anti-human IgA	Association with intestinal plasma cells	Association with secretory component	High secretion-to-serum ratio of IgA	Noncovalently linked L chains in serum IgA
Human	M > P	+	+	+	+	+ (10%)
Primates (nonhuman)	?	+	+	+	+	?
Dog	P > M	+	+	+	+	+
Cat	P > M	+	+	?	+	?
Bovine	P > M[b]	+	+	+	+	?
Goat	P > M	+	+	+	+	−[d]
Sheep	P > M	+	+	+	+	+[d]
Pig	P > M	+	+	+	+	+
Horse	P ≧ M	+	+	+	+	+ (approx. 20%)
Rabbit	P ≧ M	+	+	+	+	− NZB
Mouse	P > M	+	+	+[d]	+	+ BALB/c
Rat	M > P[b]	+[c]	+	?	+	?
Hamster	M > P	+[c]	+	?	+	?
Guinea pig	?	+	+	+	+	?
Hedgehog	M > P	+	+	?	?	?
Chicken	?	−	+	+	+	?

[a] Modified from T. B. Tomasi and H. M. Grey "Structure and function of immunoglobulin A," in *Progr. Allergy* 16:81, 1972.
[b] Conflicting data exist on the size of bovine and rat serum IgA.
[c] The hamster cross-reacts with anti-rat and anti-mouse IgA and therefore by presumption with human since these species cross-react with human.
[d] Needs confirmation.

regard to the predominance of IgA. Perhaps the most characteristic and consistent finding among the secretory systems of various species is the vast predominance in the gastrointestinal lamina propria of IgA-producing cells. Thus far this has been invariable among the species in which IgA has been definitely identified. Very recently, an immunoglobulin resembling IgA has been identified in chickens, and evidence suggests that it is also a predominant immunoglobulin in the lamina propria cells of the gastrointestinal and respiratory tracts.

ANIMAL SECRETORY SYSTEMS
SHOWING CERTAIN DIFFERENCES FROM THE HUMAN

The cow, sheep, goat, pig, and probably the horse also possess secretory systems in many ways analogous to the human's, although an important difference occurs. In these species, as in the human, secretions such as saliva and tears contain primarily IgA which is secretory in nature, i.e., 10–11S with an extra antigenic determinant presumably analogous to human SC. In bovine colostrum, much of the SC is bound to IgA while more mature milk contains a large amount of free or unattached SC. The SC of the cow (also called glycoprotein a) has physicochemical characteristics similar to human SC (see Chapter 3). Also, bovine SC binds specifically to human IgA, and conversely human SC binds to bovine IgA. Moreover, definitive evidence for homologies has been presented involving both immunological cross-reactions and N terminal sequences, indicating that bovine SC is analogous to human SC. In addition to IgA, many external secretions contain about 10–15% of IgG, predominantly 7S IgG_1 and also small amounts of IgM.

The most striking characteristic of this group which sets it apart from the human is the relative immunoglobulin content of their colostrum and milk. The predominant immunoglobulin in these secretions is 7S IgG_1, with lesser amounts of IgG_2 and IgM and only 10–15% of IgA. There is good evidence that the IgG in milk is derived in large part from serum and that transport is selective for IgG_1. In the bovine species, 7S IgG_1 remains the major immunoglobulin in mature milk, whereas in the goat the proportion of IgG to IgA decreases rapidly, and by the third or fourth day after parturition the two immunoglobulins approach each other in concentration and remain approximately equal as lactation proceeds.

ORIGIN OF IgA IN ANIMAL SECRETIONS

The origin of the immunoglobulins present in animal external secretions appears to vary both with the species and the secretion. As mentioned earlier, with the colostrum and milk of the species bovidae, there is evidence from labelling studies that the majority of the 7S IgG_1 is derived from serum, probably by selective transport. Thus, the major immunoglobulin of milk in these species is presumably synthesized in peripheral lymphoid tissues such as the spleen, bone marrow, and lymph nodes. There are also significant amounts of IgA in the colostrum and the mature milk of these species, but the origin of this has not been established. It may be derived, at least in part, from local production in the mammary gland plasma cells since bovine mammary gland organ cultures incorporate labelled amino acids into IgA, and fluorescent antibody studies have shown IgA-containing plasma cells in bovine mammary tissues. These studies, however, do not indicate the quantitative importance of local production of IgA. These same techniques applied to bovine salivary gland also demonstrate local synthesis of IgA.

In all species so far examined, the fluorescent antibody technique demonstrates that the lamina propria of the gastrointestinal tract contains large numbers of IgA cells (see for example Fig. 5-3). In some species, including the human, monkey, mouse, rat, rabbit, cow, and dog, in vitro synthesis of IgA in the GI tract has been demonstrated by organ culture experiments showing the incorporation of radiolabelled amino acids into IgA. It seems likely, therefore, that the source of the IgA present in the gastrointestinal fluids is the lamina propria IgA cells, although no direct evidence for this has been obtained and the gastrointestinal fluids from some of these species have not been directly analyzed for their relative immunoglobulin content.

Although, as shown in Table 8-1, the data in various species are far from complete, a general picture is beginning to emerge concerning the origin of the antibodies in the different secretions of various mammals. In the human as well as all other species on which data are available, the GI tract, salivary, and lacrimal glands contain a vast predominance of IgA cells. The secretions of these organs also have IgA as the major immunoglobulin class, although they also contain IgG and IgM in varying amounts. For example, GI tract fluids usually have considerably more IgG than either lacrimal or salivary secretions. It seems likely that some of the IgG and a large proportion of the IgM in these fluids are derived from local synthesis in the plasma cells seen in the lamina propria of the GI tract and in the interstitial regions of the salivary and lacrimal glands.. This thesis is verified by in vitro culture studies demonstrating synthesis of IgG and IgM in these tissues. However, the majority of the IgG in these secretions is undoubtedly derived from serum. If inflammation occurs, the proportions of the immunoglobulins are changed as a result of both increased transudation from serum as well as invasion of the organ by cells, predominantly IgG-containing, from the circulation (see Chapter 6 for more details on the origin of the various secretory immunoglobulins). The biliary system is probably very similar to the GI tract and rabbit and dog bile contains mainly IgA and a predominance of IgA cells is seen in the submucosal tissues of the gall bladder in these species. IgA has also been identified in chicken bile.

Whether the urinary and genital tracts should be included in the secretory system is uncertain for several reasons. Firstly, there is very little data in animals on the immunoglobulin content of the normal secretions from these organs. Secondly, secretions from these organs are often infected and the urine is further complicated by significant glomerular filtration of certain proteins. There is, however, good evidence in rabbits and cows that local synthesis of antibodies occurs in the genital tract, but here again the immunoglobulin class has not been determined. Local immunity in the human female genital tract is discussed in detail in Chapter 11.

REFERENCES

Goodman, M.: "Immunochemistry of the Primates and Primate Evolution," *Ann. N.Y. Acad. Sci.,* 102:219, 1962.

Vaerman, J. P.: "Comparative Immunochemistry of IgA," in *Research in Immunochemistry and Immunobiology,* ed. by J. B. G. Kwapinski, University Park Press, Baltimore, 1973.

Chapter 9

Antibody Activity

of Secretory Immunoglobulins

Secretory antibodies of the "natural" type having specificity for a variety of bacteria and viruses, as well as blood group substances, have been demonstrated in several external fluids. Although these antibodies occur in the apparent absence of the corresponding antigen, it is very likely that they result from inapparent antigenic stimulation by cross-reacting substances. This has been most clearly shown for the blood group antibodies. There is now strong evidence suggesting that blood group antibodies are formed by immunization with bacteria. For example, individuals who lack blood group B are susceptible to immunization with certain types of E. coli which contain antigens that cross-react with B substance. With other bacteria, for example α hemolytic streptococcus, SIgA antibodies are found in salivary secretions in the absence of serum antibodies, suggesting local immunization with streptococcal antigens. A summary of some of the secretory IgA antibody activities against microorganisms appearing naturally or following infection or immunization is presented in Table 9-1.

Soluble antigens such as ferritin and diphtheria toxoid, when applied to the mucous membranes, can elicit the production of secretory antibodies, again largely of the IgA class. Antibodies to soluble antigens normally ingested such as egg albumin and milk proteins can be found in GI secretions, particularly in younger children and in individuals with gastrointestinal diseases such as ulcerative colitis. In addition to antibodies to soluble antigens and microorganisms, external secretions obtained from patients with certain diseases may contain so-called "autoreactive" antibodies. For example, rheumatoid factor has been found in the saliva and urine of individuals with rheumatoid arthritis, and antinuclear factors have been detected in the secretions of patients with disseminated lupus erythematosus. Patients with pernicious anemia frequently have antibodies directed against intrinsic factor (I. F.) in their gastric fluids. Intrinsic factor is necessary for the absorption of vitamin B_{12} by the ileum and antibodies directed against I. F. can inhibit this function. It is therefore theoretically

Table 9-1

Antibody activities associated with IgA in human saliva and
intestinal secretions [a]

Antigens	Salivary	Intestinal
Blood group substances	N+	
Diphtheria toxoid	P—	
Enterococcus	N++	
Escherichia coli	N+	I++
Pneumococcus	N+	
Salmonella typhosa	N+	
Salmonella paratyphosa	P+	
Streptococcus	N++	
Tetanus toxoid	P—	
Veillonella	N++	
Vibrio cholerae	P—	I+
Coxsackie virus		I++
Echovirus		I++
Influenza virus	N+	
Influenza virus inactivated	P+	
Mumps virus	I++	
Polio virus	N+	N+
Poliovirus attenuated (Sabin)		T++
Poliovirus inactivated (Salk)	P±	P—
Rhinovirus	I+	
Candida albicans	I+	

N = normal subjects   ++ = appreciable titer
I = after infectious disease   + = low titer
P = after parenteral vaccination — = no detectable titer
T = after topical vaccination

[a] Modified from P. Brandtzaeg, in *Host Resistance to Commensal Bacteria,* edited by
T. MacPhee, Churchill Livingstone, Edinburgh, 1972.

possible that the anti-I. F. antibodies are involved in the pathogenesis of
pernicious anemia, although this has not as yet been established.

A peculiar type of IgA class antibody has been found in normal rabbit
colostrum. This antibody precipitates an organ-specific antigen derived
from the rabbit's stomach and is therefore an autoantibody. The gastric
antigen migrates more anodally than albumin, and by gel filtration has a
molecular weight of approximately 65,000. Although the function of this
system is unknown, it has been speculated that it is part of a physiological
mechanism in which the antibody, on interaction with the gastric antigen,
triggers the release of pharmacologically active substances. These in turn
enhance secretion, permeability, and/or motility of the stomach, thus aid-
ing in digestion and absorption of colostrum and perhaps serving as a
further stimulus to the newborn to feed.

VALENCE AND COMBINING AFFINITY OF SIgA ANTIBODIES

Secretory IgA and polymeric serum IgA exhibit more efficient agglutinating activity than do the corresponding serum 7S IgA or IgG-type antibodies. In fact, the IgA polymers are approximately ten times more efficient
than the corresponding monomer and are nearly as good agglutinators of
red blood cells as is 19S IgM. The greater agglutinating efficiency of polymeric IgA suggests that it has a valence greater than two. A preliminary
study of rabbit SIgA obtained by the intramammary injection of streptococcal cell wall has suggested a valence of four. In these studies, the binding
of the tritiated haptene p-nitrophenyl α, D-N-acetyl glucosaminide was
studied by equilibrium dialysis. A plot of bound versus free haptene indicated that at high haptene concentrations a limiting value of four was
reached. This suggests that the SIgA antibody molecule has four combining
sites for antigen. This is consistent with structural studies on the secretory
molecule, indicating that there are four Fab fragments per 11S IgA and
with the conformation found by electronmicroscopy (see Chapter 3). Since
each Fab unit contains one antibody-combining site, there are potentially
four such sites per 11S molecule. However, all of the potential combining
sites need not be reactive in the native molecule. For example, IgM contains ten Fab units, but only five of these combine with some macromolecular antigens. The five inactive or weak sites are probably due to
Fab units which are sterically inhibited in the native 19S IgM since, when
the Fab's are isolated following proteolysis with papain, all ten are equally
capable of combining with antigen. When an antigen such as dextran (poly-
glucose), which can be obtained in different sizes, is used in binding
studies, it can be shown that with dextran of molecular weight larger than
about 6,000, IgM antidextran antibodies have a valence of five, whereas
with lower molecular weight molecules there are ten sites available for
complexing with antigen. If similar principles apply to SIgA antibodies,
then the valence of four obtained with the haptene mentioned above may
not necessarily apply to larger antigen molecules.

As already mentioned, human SIgA is more resistant to reduction
(determined in the ultracentrifuge) than polymeric serum IgA or IgM.
This is probably due to SC which lends stability through noncovalent
associations. Rabbit colostral IgA antihaptene antibody activity is also less
sensitive to reduction than serum IgM antibody of the same specificity.
The relative resistance of SIgA antibodies to reduction, like resistance to
proteolysis, could represent a biological adaption which is advantageous to
the SIgA molecule in functioning in environments (external secretions)
which may possess significant reductive capacities.

The combining affinity of SIgA antihapten antibodies has been measured and in general is equal to those of serum IgA antibody of the same specificity. In one case, the association constant for rabbit colostral IgA antibody was approximately one log higher than the corresponding colostral IgG antibody. It is interesting that in this case, despite its high affinity, SIgA antibody did not precipitate with the antigen while the colostral IgG antibody of lesser affinity gave a good precipitation reaction under identical conditions. The reason for this difference is unknown but probably involves the solubility characteristics of the respective antigen/antibody complexes.

Another indication of the combining affinity of antibodies synthesized in the secretory system comes from studies of mouse myeloma proteins. Mouse myelomas can be induced in an appropriate strain of mice by the intraperitoneal injection of an irritant such as mineral oil. About 70% of the myelomas so induced are of the IgA class, and it has been suggested that the high incidence of IgA proteins occurs because they arise from cells of intestinal origin. The fact that many of the myelomas have antibody-like activity against bacterial antigens of enteric origin is consistent with this hypothesis. About 10% of these myelomas also bind nitrophenyl ligands with affinities which are in the same range as conventionally produced antibodies. One well-studied murine IgA protein (MOPC-315) has a binding constant for dinitrophenyl-L-lysine (DNP) of $1:6 \times 10^7\ M^{-1}$. The DNP binding probably represents a cross-reaction in which the primary antigen is a substance such as menadione (vitamin K) which is normally found in the mouse GI tract. Very few human IgA proteins have been found with DNP binding activity (in one study, only 1 out of 90), and there is no evidence that the majority of human IgA myelomas arise in the secretory system. An exception may be the rare IgA myeloma in which the initial lesion is restricted to the gastrointestinal tract, and to the author's knowledge, none of these proteins have been shown to have antibody activity.

IMMUNOLOGICAL MEMORY IN THE SECRETORY SYSTEM

Very little data are available concerning the persistence of immunity in the secretory system. It is known that following oral immunization with cholera, both in experimental animals and in humans, gastrointestinal immunity appears to be short-lived, on the order of a few weeks to a few months. In experimental guinea pig conjunctivitis with a trachoma-like organism, immunity to reinfection in the eye persists for only about a month. Also, following topical immunization of the nasopharynx with killed polio or influenza vaccine, antibodies can be detected in respiratory secretions for about 3–6 months, although in one recent study employing high doses of the vaccine, significant titers against influenza were found as long as one year following immunization.

Long-lived immunity has, however, been recorded following immunization with live attenuated polio virus with persistence of essentially unchanged titers of antipolio antibodies in nasopharyngeal secretions for as long as three years following immunization. Why the polio antibody titers persist unchanged for such a long period is not fully understood, but there may be a basic difference between live versus inactivated antigens in this regard. It seems likely that with live vaccines there may be persistence of viral antigen in an as yet unrecognized and unculturable form. It has not been excluded, however, that the observed differences in persistence of antibody between live and killed vaccines are not simply a result of antigenic dose. It might be expected that the dose of antigen would be considerably greater in the case of live viruses which actually colonize and replicate in the mucosal area where they elicit their response.

There seems to be little in the way of immunological memory in the secretory system. This statement is based primarily on the observation that, following immunization with certain antigens such as inactivated polio vaccine, the antibody titers in nasal secretions after a second immunization appear at about the same time and reach nearly identical levels as following a primary stimulus. Although more data with different antigens are certainly needed, these findings are consistent with other evidence in animals, suggesting that there may be little in the way of a memory effect with the secretory IgA antibody response.

Plasma cells are, for the most part, end cells, i.e., once a lymphoid cell has differentiated into a plasma cell, further cell divisions do not occur. Pertinent to the question of immunological memory is the life span of the end-stage plasma cell. Dr. Carlos Mattioli and I have measured the half-life of the intestinal plasma cell of the mouse by the following technique. Mice were given daily injections of tritiated thymidine between days 15 and 35 after birth. During this three-week period, there is a rapid proliferation of cells in the lamina propria, and by day 35 essentially 100% of the plasma cells have labelled nuclei resulting from incorporation of thymidine into nuclear DNA. Labelled IgA cells could be recognized by a technique which combines autoradiography and immunofluorescence (see Fig. 9-1). By quantitating cells and following the decline in the number of labelled IgA cells after the discontinuance of thymidine, the mean half-life of an intestinal IgA cell was calculated to be 4.8 days. Thus, there must be a continued renewal of plasma cells from lymphoid precursors and significant numbers of long-lived plasma cells do not exist.

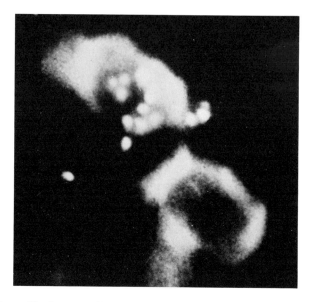

Fig. 9-1. High-magnification view of two IgA plasma cells in the intestinal lamina propria of a mouse injected with tritiated thymidine (TTH) during the neonatal period. The plasma cell on the top shows many silver grains over the nucleus. The other plasma cell is unlabelled. Mouse killed 10 days after the last TTH injection. Combined immunofluorescentautoradiograph technique. The half-life of IgA cells was estimated from the rate of disappearance of tritiated cells to be about 5 days.

REFERENCES

Eisen, H. N., M. C. Michaelides, B. J. Underdown, E. P. Schulenburg, and E. S. Simms: "Myeloma Proteins with Antihapten Antibody Activity," *Fed. Proc.*, 29:78, 1970.

Ishizaka, K., T. Ishizaka, E. H. Lee, and H. H. Fudenberg: "Immunochemical Properties of Human γA Isohemagglutinin. I. Comparisons with γG- and γM-globulin Antibodies," *J. Immunol.*, 95:197, 1965.

Mattioli, C. A., and T. B. Tomasi: "The Life Span of IgA Plasma Cells from the Mouse Intestine," *J. Exp. Med.*, 138:452, 1973.

Potter, M.: "Mouse IgA Myeloma Proteins that Bind Polysaccharide Antigens of Enterobacterial Origin," *Fed. Proc.*, 29:85, 1970.

Taubman, M. A., and R. J. Genco: "Induction and Properties of Rabbit Secretory γA Antibody Directed to Group A Streptococcal Carbohydrate," *Immunochemistry*, 8:1137, 1971.

Chapter 10

Mechanism of Biological Action
of Secretory Antibodies

The mucous membranes are of vital importance in protecting the host, since it is here that potential microbial pathogens and toxic agents make their first contact with the host. The mucous membrane defenses may either prevent implantation or eliminate the agent following an initial successful colonization. In the case of nonviable toxins, preventing their absorption may be the key defense function.

The mechanisms by which mucous membranes exert their protective functions are complex and in large part incompletely understood. Table 10-1 lists some of the many factors which may cooperatively interact to maintain mucous membrane defenses. This chapter is concerned with specific as opposed to nonspecific factors and will focus exclusively on the role of the secretory immune system. The secretory system has been called the "first line of defense," while factors such as IgG-type antibodies derived from the circulation are referred to as "second line." Second-line factors are often called into play at mucous membrane surfaces once the agent has implanted and become sufficiently established to induce a local inflammatory reaction. The interplay of first- and second-line specific factors along with nonspecific factors may then result in the containment and/or elimination of the pathogenic agent. The protective role of the secretory immune system, which includes both B and T cell-mediated components, is best understood for viral infections, but has more recently been extended to bacterial systems and to nonviable agents such as inhaled and ingested antigens.

Viral Neutralization

Animal studies and experiments involving the relative efficiency of local versus systemic immunization in several human diseases suggest that secretory antibodies may function to protect mucous membranes against invasion by potentially pathogenic viruses. It is also known that antibodies

93

Table 10-1

Factors involved in host protection against infectious agents. Some of the possibilities for interactions or cooperation are indicated by arrows.[a]

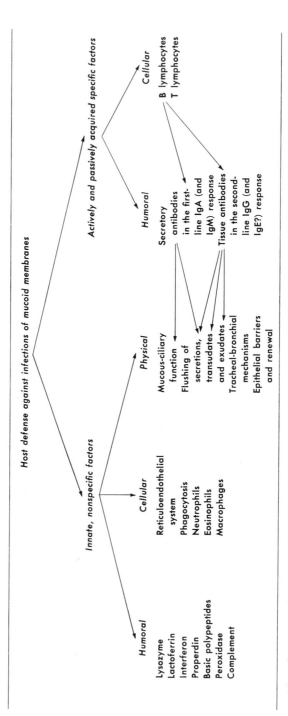

Host defense against infections of mucoid membranes

Innate, nonspecific factors

Actively and passively acquired specific factors

Humoral

Lysozyme
Lactoferrin
Interferon
Properdin
Basic polypeptides
Peroxidase
Complement

Cellular

Reticuloendothelial system
Phagocytosis
Neutrophils
Eosinophils
Macrophages

Physical

Mucous-ciliary function
Flushing of secretions, transudates and exudates
Tracheal-bronchial mechanisms
Epithelial barriers and renewal

Humoral

Secretory antibodies in the first-line IgA (and IgM) response
Tissue antibodies in the second-line IgG (and IgE?) response

Cellular

B lymphocytes
T lymphocytes

[a] Data from P. Brandtzaeg, in *Host Resistance to Commensal Bacteria*, edited by T. MacPhee, Churchill Livingstone, Edinburgh, 1972.

of several classes are capable of neutralizing viruses and inhibiting their growth in vitro. Viral neutralization may occur in the absence of complement fixation (as with IgA-type antibodies), but with those classes capable of fixation, neutralization may involve the participation of at least some of the components of the complement system. For example, herpes simplex virus sensitized with IgM antibody is neutralized by the addition of the first and fourth components of complement, and the subsequent addition of other components does not enhance neutralization. Whether there is sufficient complement in external secretions to support a lytic reaction is unknown. The only component which has been definitely shown to be produced locally in the secretory system is C1, which is synthesized by the gut epithelial cells. However, since macrophages apparently are the cellular source of many of the complement proteins (exclusive of C1), it is possible that these cell types, which are relatively abundant in secretory organs such as the respiratory and gastrointestinal tracts, could be a significant source of complement in external secretions. More work is vitally needed in this area particularly in regard to the alternate pathway components in various secretions.

Viral neutralization has been directly demonstrated with SIgA antibodies, and evidence is available that such antibodies acting at the mucosal surface can prevent implantation and therefore colonization at the portal of entry. This could constitute an important mucosal protective mechanism and will be discussed in detail in Chapter 11.

ANTIBACTERIAL ACTIVITY

Complement fixation

Although a role for SIgA antibodies in resistance to viral infections seems very likely, the mechanism by which secretory immunoglobulins exert a protective effect against bacteria is more uncertain. It is generally believed that killing of bacteria by antibody involves the lysis of the bacterial cell and that this requires the fixation of complement. There is now ample evidence that IgA antibodies, both those in serum and secretions, do not fix complement, at least by classical mechanisms. However, it has been suggested that SIgA antibodies together with complement and lysozyme (an enzyme) have a lytic capacity for certain types of E. coli. In this system, which needs confirmation, antibody, complement, and lysozyme are all required for lysis of the bacterial cell. Whether such a mechanism has an important antibacterial function in native secretions has not been established.

Antibodies against many of the bacteria which are commonly found on mucous membranes (such as streptococci) and those frequently associated with human diseases (such as pneumococci) do not inhibit the growth of these organisms in the absence of other factors such as complement or phagocytic cells. It is not yet known whether secretory antibodies of the IgG and IgM class, which are capable of complement fixation and opsonization in vitro, are able to kill bacteria in vivo in native secretions. One of the problems complicating an evaluation of the role of antibodies in resistance to bacterial infections is the presence in many secretions of non-immune factors; for example, the enzyme peroxidase found in milk and saliva has important antibacterial properties.

Statements regarding the inability of IgA antibodies to fix complement stem largely from studies using either heat or bis-diazo-benzidine aggregated IgA myeloma proteins. In these experiments, the ability of aggregated IgA proteins to utilize complement through the classical scheme involving the sequential fixation of C1, C4, C2, C3, C5–C9 is shown in Fig. 10-1. The classical sequence is initiated by the interaction of antibody with Clq, and apparently IgA aggregated in this manner does not contain or expose the appropriate receptors to initiate this reaction. The alternate or shunt pathway of complement fixation does not utilize the early components (C1, C4, and C2) but rather the properdin system and activation begins directly with C3. A number of nonimmunoglobulin substances have been found to activate the C3 shunt, including bacterial lipopolysaccharides

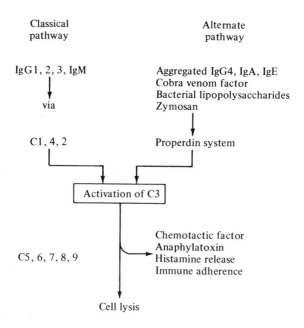

Fig. 10-1. Complement fixation: Comparison of the classical and alternate pathways.

(such as E. coli endotoxin), inulin, and cobra venom. Most important, certain immunoglobulin classes which do not fix complement through the classical scheme have been found to be capable of initiating the C3 shunt. These include guinea pig γl and human IgE, IgG_4 and serum, and secretory IgA. Selective depletion of components of the alternate pathway from human serum reduces the bactericidal activity of the serum for certain organisms such as E. coli. This pathway may therefore have important antibacterial functions, and it is possible that IgA antibody directed against bacteria could fix complement in the presence of the components of the shunt pathway. Despite the above, alternate pathway activation has not been directly demonstrated for IgA antibodies (other than aggregated myeloma proteins), and there have been no published studies to date as to whether the components of the shunt pathway are present in external secretions in sufficient concentrations to support antibacterial activities.

Opsonization

It has been suggested that IgA antibodies may exert an antibacterial effect through opsonization (promoting phagocytosis). It is known that phagocytosis by macrophages can occur in the absence of complement. Very recent work suggests that the C3 shunt may also be active in opsonization. For example, heat labile opsonic activity in human serum for Escherichia coli, Proteus mirabilis, Staphylococcus aureus, and Diplococcus pneumonia can be effected through the alternate pathway. Thus, IgA antibodies together with the components of the shunt pathway could conceivably promote the ingestion of organisms and subsequent killing by phagocytic cells. However, when one critically examines the experiments in which specific SIgA antibodies were tested for their opsonizing activity, discordant results are found. In general, when highly pure preparations of SIgA antibodies against gram-negative organisms have been tested for opsonization, no activity has been obtained. For example, in one study in which positive opsonization by IgA preparations for enteric bacteria was reported, further investigations by the same worker with more purified preparations obtained with the aid of immunoadsorbents showed that contamination with very small amounts of highly active IgM-type opsonins was responsible. The absence of specific receptors on human macrophages which are cytophilic for IgA is consistent with the lack of opsonization by IgA antibody. In contradiction to the studies with bacteria, evidence has been obtained which suggests that human SIgA anti-blood-group-A antibodies will opsonize red cells for phagocytosis by human macrophages. Thus, the whole question of an opsonizing activity for IgA should be studied in more depth with particular emphasis on differences between antigens and opsonizing ability of various cell types and on the possible participation of the C3 shunt. If opsonization is eventually shown to be a significant protective mechanism, it seems more likely that it would occur in the interstitial areas just below the mucosa rather than in the lumenal contents where phagocytic cells are few in number.

Inhibition of bacterial adherence to epithelial surfaces

It seems likely that for a bacteria to colonize a mucous surface it must first adhere to the outer (lumenal) surface of the mucous membrane. Bacteria that do not adhere would presumably be swept away in the bathing fluid, i.e., by swallowing, by the peristaltic activity of the small intestine, or by the cilia of the respiratory tract. Only if bacterial replication was very rapid compared with the wash-out time of a continuous flow system such as the intestinal tract would sufficient numbers of microorganisms accumulate in the lumen to produce pathological effects. On the other hand, bacteria that were able to adhere firmly to the mucosa would have, other things being equal, more time to proliferate locally and, therefore, would reach larger numbers. In certain bacterial systems, for example in the production of dental caries (see below), it is a requirement that the bacteria physically attach to the surface of the tooth in order to produce a cavity. Thus, of great interest are studies in two bacterial systems which suggest that SIgA antibodies are effective in preventing adherence of bacteria to epithelial cells. One involves inhibition by salivary antibodies of the absorption of cariogenic streptococci to human buccal epithelial cells; the other involves a reduction in the absorption of Vibrio cholerae to the intestinal mucosa by SIgA antibodies.

Recent studies from the Forsyth Dental Center in Boston have demonstrated that SIgA fractions isolated from normal parotid saliva contain antibodies which are capable of inhibiting the adherence of certain strains of Streptococci to buccal epithelial cells. In these experiments, the Streptococci are first coated with the isolated SIgA preparations. The bacteria are then washed and incubated with isolated buccal epithelial cells obtained by scraping the oral mucosa. After the cells are washed to remove nonspecifically adsorbed bacteria, the number of adherent bacteria per cell are counted by light microscopy and compared with the number of bacteria bound in controls having no antibody (see Fig. 10-2). Some typical data are illustrated in Table 10-2. The inhibition is specific in that only those

---

Fig. 10-2. Adherence of streptococcus salivarius to buccal epithelial cells. (a) Cheek epithelial cells incubated with S. salivarius. (b) same as (a) except streptococci incubated with SIgA antibodies specific for the organism prior to exposure to epithelial cells. The figure illustrates that the specific antibodies inhibit the attachment of the bacteria to the surface of the epithelial cell. (Data from R. J. Gibbons and J. van Haute, *Infection and Immunity*, 3:567, 1971.) See also Table 10-2 for quantitative counts of adherent bacteria.

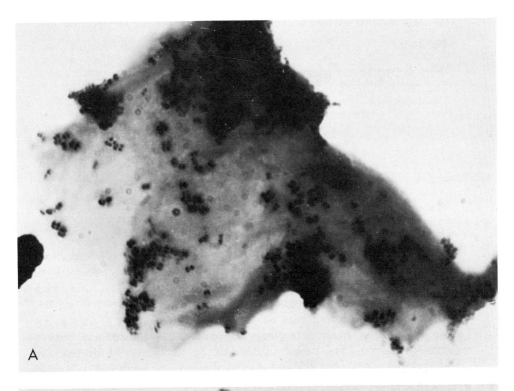

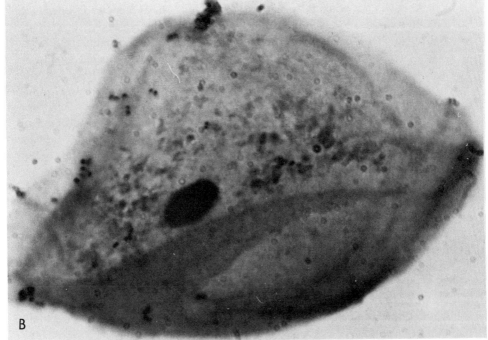

Table 10-2

Inhibition of adherence of S. salivarius to human buccal epithelial
cells by parotid fluid SIgA [a]

Prior treatment of bacteria	Adherence (% of control [b])
Buffer (control)	100
Parotid fluid	56
65 μg. of SIgA	24
SIgA + anti-IgA	98

[a] Data from R. C. Williams and R. J. Gibbons, Science, 177:697, 1972.

[b] $\dfrac{\text{Number of bacteria per epithelial cell test system}}{\text{Number of bacteria per epithelial cell in control}} \times 100$

strains of streptococci which are agglutinated by the salivary SIgA fractions are inhibited, indicating that a nonspecific salivary inhibitor is not involved. The fractions having an inhibitory capacity contain only IgA, and prior treatment of these fractions with anti-IgA removes the inhibitory activity. Although in these experiments evidence was obtained that SIgA was inhibitory, it seems likely that other immunoglobulin classes may behave similarly. For example, rabbit antisera to the M antigen of streptococci inhibited the adherence of Streptococcus pyogenes to epithelial cells, and the antibodies are of the IgG type.

A new and potentially important mechanism of action of intestinal coproantibodies has been advanced by R. Freter and his associates in Michigan. They have found that guinea pigs previously immunized with Vibrio cholerae so as to induce coproantibodies were protected against a subsequent oral challenge with the live organism. A similar type of local protection was demonstrated in several other cholera models, including the suckling rabbit and isolated loops of adult rabbit small intestine. Interestingly, protection in immune animals is not associated with a reduction in the overall growth rate of the Vibrio; however, the bacteria tended to remain free in the lumen and the numbers invading the mucous membrane were greatly reduced. Subsequent studies attempting to elucidate the mechanisms showed that sera from immune rabbits containing antibodies against the cholera organisms inhibited attachment of the bacteria to the intestinal mucosa of in vivo isolated loops or to slices of rabbit ileum in vitro. Some typical data from these experiments are shown in Table 10-3. These effects were specific in that an antiserum specific for Salmonella inhibited the attachment of Salmonella and not the Vibrio. The experiments illustrated in Table 10-3 employed whole antisera, and the inhibition of adherence was undoubtedly due to antibodies of the IgG type. More recent studies with isolated intestinal SIgA anticholera antibodies have shown a similar inhibition of adsorption. These data suggest that locally synthesized SIgA and

Table 10-3[a]

Effect of antibody on the adsorption and multiplication of bacteria on slices of rabbit ileum.[b]

	Cholera No. of bacteria/slice $\times 10^3$ Incubation		Salmonella No. of bacteria/slice $\times 10^3$ Incubation	
Antisera	Before	After	Before	After
Normal rabbit serum	1,785	5,325	90	1,635
Anti V. cholerae antiserum	210	360	105	1,725

[a] Data from R. Freter, *Infection and Immunity*, 2:556, 1970.
[b] Slices (1 $\times$ 2 cm) dipped into a mixture of the two bacteria plus antiserum or normal serum. Number of bacteria per slice counted before and after incubation at 37°C for one hour in presence of whole normal or anti-cholera rabbit serum.

antibodies derived from serum may both participate in mucosal antibacterial activity.

Two hypotheses may be considered to explain the observed inhibition of adsorption of bacteria. First, antibodies may directly inhibit the adherence of the organisms to the surface epithelium. Alternatively, the initial adsorption may be normal, but the subsequent growth of the organisms on the mucosa may be inhibited. Since the total number of organisms in intestinal loops is the same in the presence and absence of antibody, inhibition must be restricted to those organisms adsorbed and not those in the lumen. Experiments by Freter have clearly demonstrated that both mechanisms occur. Antibody significantly decreases the adsorption of heat-killed as well as live bacteria to the mucosal surface in the ileal loop model. Since antibodies (with complement) were unable to lyse the heat-killed cholera organism in vitro, it was concluded that they had a direct effect on adsorption. An even greater effect was noted when live organisms were used and the number of viable organisms were determined before and after incubation of slices of rabbit ileum (see Table 10-3). No inhibition of growth was noted when filter paper or mucosal scrapings instead of slices of ileum were used. Also, the addition of the organism directly to the antiserum did not inhibit their growth when compared to that in normal serum. These data, taken together, suggest that the viable mucosa supplies an accessory substance(s) which, acting in concert with antibody, exerts an antibacterial effect. Substances such as lysozyme, lactoferrin, and complement have been suggested as possible ancillary factors. It should be remembered that the slices and loops used in these studies contain cell types other than epithelial cells such as polymorphs and macrophages, and the participation of these cells or factors secreted by them should be investigated in future studies.

The biological properties of the different classes of rabbit anti-Vibrio-cholera antibodies have been carefully studied by Rowley and his associates in Adelaide, Australia as shown in Table 10-4. These workers have demon-

Table 10-4

Biological properties of rabbit IgG, IgM, and IgA classes of
V. cholerae antibody [a]

Immunoglobulin	HA	HL	VIB	OPS	PD50
IgG	1–0	1–0	170	600	6
IgM	9–0	22	8,000	17,000	6
SIgA	2–0	< 0–3	< 30	90	13

Values are reciprocals of greatest dilution of a somatic antibody preparation achieving desired effect.
HA = hemagglutination with 569B Vibrio cholerae LPS coated sheep red blood cells
HL = haemolysis of the same red cells in the presence of fresh guinea pig serum
VIB = in vitro killing of 569B Vibrio cholerae in the presence of fresh guinea pig serum
OPS = intraperitoneal phagocytic assay (young adult mice)
PD50 = infant mouse protection assay
SIgA isolated from colostrum

[a] Data from E. J. Steele, W. Chaicumpa, and D. Rowley, *J. Inf. Dis.*, 130:93, 1974.

strated that although SIgA antibodies against the somatic antigen of the Vibrio fail to kill organisms in vitro and do not facilitate phagocytosis, they nevertheless are highly potent in protecting against a challenge with the live organisms. In the mouse protection assay employed in these studies, infant mice which are highly susceptible to cholera are fed the live organisms which have been premixed with varying amounts of the different classes of antibodies. The dilution of the antibody preparation necessary to reduce mortality to 50% is then calculated and expressed as the PD50. Thus the higher the PD50 (last column of Table 10-4), the more potent the antibody preparation in protection. The mechanism by which SIgA protects in this system has not been established, but a reasonable possibility is that the antibody coating the organism prevents adherence to the gut epithelium.

The antibacterial system discussed above would interfere with the early phase of an infection by preventing the establishment of significant numbers of organisms to effect a critical population size. In the natural situation, this system would be functionally integrated with other defense mechanisms. For example, it is known that the growth of an invading pathogen may be markedly reduced by the antagonistic action of the normal bacterial flora. Thus, nonimmune mechanisms working in conjunction with mucosal-associated antibody may constitute a particularly effective first-line defense reaction.

In regard to the normal flora, it is known that the bacteria present in human saliva are coated with SIgA. This coating may suppress adherence as suggested by the observation that epithelial cells scraped from human cheeks contain only 10–15 bacteria per cell, whereas epithelial cells treated in vitro with Streptococci which do not have antibody on their surfaces absorb several hundred bacteria within a few minutes. There may therefore be a delicate balance between the various partially suppressed indigenous microorganisms comprising the normal flora. The observed fluctuations in the serotypes and phagetypes of bacteria normally colonizing mucous surfaces could result at least partly from the suppressing effect of antibody. For example, the absence of immunity to a new serotype of E. coli would allow it to colonize and outgrow existing serotypes. Eventually, the antibody response would again establish an equilibrium. Thus, relatively minute amounts of new organisms may be able to gain a foothold and whether or not they become a more permanent member of the flora would depend upon a number of factors, including the ability to stimulate adherence-inhibiting antibodies.

LIMITING ABSORPTION OF NONVIABLE ANTIGENS

The gastrointestinal tract of newborn animals of many species is freely permeable to ingested macromolecules. Each species has a characteristic time period over which its GI tract is highly permeable, varying from 2–3 days in the cow to 18–20 days in mice and rats (see also Chapter 5). In man, the newborn gastrointestinal tract is generally believed to be essentially impermeable to macromolecules, and it is frequently stated that very little if any absorption of intact proteins including antibodies occurs in the immediate postpartum period. However, when one examines the literature carefully, it is clear that in many species small but significant amounts of antigenically intact macromolecules can be absorbed through the adult gastrointestinal epithelium (see also Chapter 5). For example, studies have been performed in sensitized guinea pigs showing absorption of sufficient amounts of antigenically intact material from the adult intestinal tract to elicit an immediate-type skin reaction. Another example is the serum antibody response which regularly follows the oral ingestion of antigens such as bovine serum or egg albumin. An indication of a systemic antibody response in these experiments is the finding of antibody-containing cells by both the fluorescent and Jerne plaque techniques in peripheral lymphoid tissues such as the spleen. That these cells were stimulated in situ by absorbed antigen rather than having migrated from the gut is suggested by the finding that the splenic plaques produced specific antibody of the IgM and IgG types, while the intestinal cells were restricted to

IgA. The distribution of antibodies to egg albumin in the human also suggests that lymphoid cells, in both the gastrointestinal tract and the peripheral lymphoid tissues, contain an antibody to this naturally ingested antigen. It appears, therefore, that the adult of many species including man is capable of absorbing small but significant amounts of antigens. Moreover, as illustrated by the egg-white studies, the human gastrointestinal tract is capable of forming antibodies against food antigens.

Conditions which seem to favor the absorption of intact macromolecules include not only the small size of the antigen, but also inflammation of the gastrointestinal tract. For example, diarrhea from any cause results in an increased absorption of egg-white antigens. The introduction of inhibitors of proteolytic enzymes into the intestinal tract also favors absorption since the great bulk of absorption occurs in the stomach and upper intestine which contains several proteolytic enzymes. Although the data are scanty, it seems likely that younger animals (first few months or year of life) have a somewhat more permeable GI tract than adults. This may also be true in man since studies of serum antibody levels directed against bovine milk antigens have consistently demonstrated a significantly higher frequency and titers in children (particularly under the age of 12) than in adults. The higher titers in children are presumably the result of a greater absorption of milk antigens.

Among the explanations offered to elucidate the progressive decline in the permeability of the GI tract with age is an association with the maturation of the secretory system. One of the lines of evidence favoring this is the finding that individuals who are selectively deficient in IgA have a high incidence (about 75%) of high titers of antibody against various bovine milk antigens. Particularly striking is the observation that IgA-deficient individuals frequently have large amounts of precipitating IgG antibody in their sera against bovine IgM, whereas antibodies against this antigen are very rarely found in normal children or adults. The ability of IgA-deficient individuals to absorb such a large macromolecule in amounts sufficient to stimulate high titers of serum antibody may be related to their inability to form local IgA antibodies, which blocks absorption. That intestinal immunity (presumably antibody-mediated) can influence absorption has been demonstrated in animals orally immunized with soluble antigens such as bovine serum albumin and horseradish peroxidase. Employing inverted gut sacs of jejunum or ileum, the transport of the I^{125}-labelled proteins can be studied in immunized versus control animals. As shown in Table 10-5, a significant decrease in uptake was noted in immunized intestines compared with controls, and the inhibition of absorption is specific for the immunizing antigen.

Although the role of the secretory system in regulating absorption of nonviable antigens is potentially very important, it should be emphasized

Table 10-5

Effect of prior immunization of rats on the intestinal uptake
of protein absorption of radiolabelled (I^{125}) proteins studied
using everted gut sacs [a]

Oral immunization with:	Protein absorption of:	Absorption (% of control)	
		Jejunum	Ileum
BSA	HRP^{125}	99	97
(Bovine serum	BSA^{125}	50	70
albumin)			
HRP	BSA^{125}	80	110
(Horseradish	HRP^{125}	38	33
peroxidase)			

[a] Data from W. A. Walker, K. J. Isselbacher, and K. J. Block, *Science*, 177:608, 1972.

that other factors such as proteolytic enzymes and the physical barrier of
the mucosal epithelium are also of prime importance. If the secretory
system does have a role in regulating absorption as the above data suggest,
it seems likely that it is a modulating effect which will be restricted to the
relatively small amounts, which escape other limiting mechanisms.

IMMEDIATE-TYPE HYPERSENSITIVITY REACTIONS

IgE

IgE is known to be an important mediator of immediate-type hypersensitivity reactions. This immunoglobulin is capable of fixing to human
skin and is responsible for the wheal and erythemia-type skin reactions
that occur on injection of allergins into the skin of appropriately sensitive
individuals. In the passive transfer of hypersensitivity to normal individuals (the so-called PK reaction), it is the IgE in the serum derived from
the allergic patient which transfers the skin reactivity to the normal individual.

IgE is present in high concentrations in the respiratory and gastrointestinal secretions relative to serum and it appears that IgE, like IgA,
may be synthesized in large part in secretory sites. It is not surprising,
therefore, that IgE antibodies directed against several allergins, particularly ragweed, have been identified in the secretions of sensitive individuals.
In this regard, electron microscope studies employing ferritin-tagged anti-
IgE have demonstrated IgE on the surface of circulating basophils. When
an isolated IgE myeloma protein is added in vitro to basophils or to tissue
mast cells, it is "cytophilic" for these cells and it can be shown that the

Fc fragment is required for surface attachment. Treatment of basophils which have adsorbed the IgE myeloma with anti-IgE results in histamine release. Specific anti-ragweed antibodies of the IgE type will also adsorb to and sensitize basophils derived from a nonallergic individual. These in vitro sensitized cells will then release histamine on exposure to ragweed antigen. In view of these findings, it seems likely that IgE antibodies fixed to the surface of mast cells located in the submucosal areas of the upper respiratory tract, upon interaction with the allergin, result in the release of the pharmacologically active agents such as histamine which are responsible for the allergic symptoms. Some key relationships in immediate-type allergies are schematically depicted in Figure 10-3.

Certain types of so-called "extrinsic" asthma may also be mediated by IgE-type antibodies locally synthesized in pulmonary tissues. In this case, the major symptoms, dyspnea and wheezing, are caused by narrowing of the bronchi induced by mediators such as histamine, slow reactive substances (SRS), and kinins. However, in the majority of cases of chronic asthma, a definite antigen has not been identified and most workers doubt that hypersensitivity reactions are primarily involved in these cases. It should also be pointed out that certain cases of allergic asthma may be mediated at least in part by antibodies other than IgE. For example, when

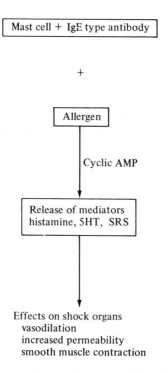

Fig. 10-3. Postulated sequence in the development of IgE-mediated hypersensitivity reactions.

patients with bronchopulmonary aspergillosis are challenged with an aerosol of the mold, an immediate attack of asthma occurs which is probably mediated by IgE. The attack usually subsides in 10–20 minutes but is followed in 5 or 6 hours by a second, often more severe, episode. Although it has not been definitely proven, it seems likely that the latter attacks are mediated by an IgG antibody and that the immune complexes (IgG + mold antigen) induce a pulmonary-arthus-type reaction. In patients with late reactions, IgG-type precipitins have been demonstrated in the serum and this is probably the source of the pulmonary antibody, although some local synthesis may also occur.

Similar reactions may occur in the gastrointestinal tract in certain cases of milk and food allergies. However, IgE-type antibodies specific for an antigen have not been clearly identified in gastrointestinal secretions. Locally synthesized IgE antibodies may have an important function in the so-called self-cure reactions which follow some parasitic infestations. It is known that expulsion of certain parasites from the gastrointestinal tract is preceded by a striking increase in the number of tissue mast cells in the lamina propria. This is followed by degranulation and release of mediators which in turn cause an increase in gastrointestinal motility with the expulsion of the parasites. Although it has been suggested that IgE antibodies directed against parasitic antigens are responsible for the mast cell degranulation reaction, this has not yet been definitely established. There is some conflict among workers in the field regarding the role played by IgE. For example, some workers have suggested that IgE antibodies play a secondary role and function primarily to increase capillary permeability, thereby promoting transudation of serum IgG antibodies which inactivate the parasite. Further investigations in this area are needed to clarify the role of IgE and other locally produced antibodies in parasitic reactions.

Blocking activity

Parotid saliva and nasal wash IgA and IgG levels are comparable in atopic (allergic) and normal age-matched controls. Thus, there is no evidence of an exocrine immunoglobulin deficiency in atopic individuals that might allow an increased adsorption of natural allergens across the respiratory mucosa. However, IgA-deficient patients do have an increased incidence of respiratory allergies, and here an enhanced adsorption of inhaled antigens could play a role in this selected group of patients.

Nasal secretions have been found to contain "blocking" antibodies and these are partly of the IgA class. Specimens from both normal and allergic individuals contain blocking activity against ragweed and grass pollens, but not against an unrelated antigen such as pitressin to which the subjects have not been exposed. However, since there appears to be little relationship between clinical allergy and the presence of these antibodies, their significance seems doubtful. Another antibody which has been described in the saliva of the ragweed allergic but not normal individuals fixes to isolated strips of monkey ileum in vitro and sensitizes them to contraction on subsequent exposure to antigen (positive Schultz-Dale reaction). This antibody is of the IgA class and may be present in the saliva in the absence of IgE (skin-sensitizing) antibody. Its role in ragweed allergy is unknown.

The question of blocking antibodies either of the IgG or IgA class in the secretions of allergic individuals is an important one and much more work is needed. It seems logical that if an antibody is to effectively block a mucosal allergic reaction, it should do so before the antigen reaches the tissue mast cells with their surface-fixed IgE antibody. Thus, a high concentration of blocking activity in the secretions and in the interstitial fluid surrounding the mast cells may be critical to effective blocking action. Several groups are presently experimenting with methods of desensitization (such as topical application of small amounts of antigen) in an attempt to elicit the local synthesis of secretory blocking antibodies.

REFERENCES

Brandtzaeg, P.: "Local Formation and Transport of Immunoglobulins Related to the Oral Cavity," in *Host Resistance to Commensal Bacteria,* ed. by T. MacPhee, Churchill Livingstone, Edinburgh, 1972.

Buckley, R. H., and S. C. Dees: "Correlation of Milk Precipitins with IgA Deficiency," *New Eng. J. Med.,* 281:465, 1969.

Eddie, D. S., M. L. Schulkind, and J. B. Robbins: "The Isolation nad Biologic Activities of Purified Secretory IgA and IgG Anti-Salmonella Typhimurium 'O' Antibodies from Rabbit Intestinal Fluid and Colostrum," *J. Immunol.,* 106:181, 1971.

Fubara, E. S., and R. Freter: "Source and Protective Function of Coproantibodies in Intestinal Disease," *Amer. J. Clin. Nutr.,* 25:1357, 1972.

Ishizaka, K.: "Chemistry and Biology of Immunoglobulin E," in *The Antigens,* ed. by M. Sela, Academic Press, Inc., New York, 1973, p. 479.

McCombs, R. P.: "Diseases Due to Immunologic Reactions in the Lungs," *New Eng. J. Med.,* 286:1186 and 286:1245, 1972.

Ruddy, S., I. Gigli, and K. F. Austen: "The Complement System of Man," *New Eng. J. Med.,* 287:489; 287:545; 287:592, and 287:642, 1972.

Williams, R. C., and R. J. Gibbons: "Inhibition of Bacterial Adherence by Secretory Immunoglobulin A: A Mechanism of Antigen Disposal," *Science,* 177:697, 1972.

Chapter 11

Role of the Secretory System in

Protection and Immunization

Against Infection

In the introduction to Chapter 10, a brief summary was presented of the various factors involved in the host's defenses at the mucous membrane level. It was pointed out that the IgA system may serve as a first line of defense against infections, and some of the specific mechanisms by which IgA may exert this function were discussed in some detail. Table 11-1 summarizes some of the mechanisms involved and again points out

Table 11-1

Hypothetical mucosal defense mechanisms mediated by immunoglobulins

First-line defenses [a]	Second-line defenses [b]
1. Trapping of organism at mucous surface	1. Viral neutralization
2. Coating of organism and inhibition of adherence to mucosa	2. Lysis of bacteria
3. Viral neutralization	3. Toxin neutralization
4. Toxin neutralization	4. Opsonization
5. Lysis of bacteria	5. Immune complex formation with complement fixation resulting in inflammation, immune adherence, opsonization, chemotaxis, and anaphylatoxin
6. Opsonization	

[a] Primarily IgA but also other locally synthesized immunoglobulins. Lysis of bacteria and opsonization, if they occur at all, are mediated by immunoglobulins other than IgA.
[b] Primarily IgG from serum.

the concept of the first- and second-line defenses. In actuality, this separation, although conceptually useful, is somewhat artificial since with a given agent the various factors listed in both categories may be intermeshed and may be involved to different degrees at various stages in the infection. In general, the first-line defenses are concerned with the prevention of

109

infection. If specific antibodies are already present either as a result of previous exposure to the agent or immunization and the dose of the organism is not too large, the infection will be terminated by one or more of the mechanisms listed in Table 11-1. Large numbers of organisms may exceed the capacity of existing immune (and other) mechanisms, but the secondary immune response is able to eliminate the agent before sufficient numbers of organisms are generated to produce clinically significant disease. In the absence of secretory antibody, whether an organism will produce disease will depend on several factors including the size of the inoculum, its ability to overcome nonimmune defenses and proliferation locally, and its virulence. Once an organism penetrates the mucous membrane and comes into contact with existing specific antibody and/or cells in the interstitial regions of the mucous membrane, then the various factors listed under second-line defenses in Table 11-1, along with other non-immune mechanisms, are brought into play. Particularly important is the development of immune complexes which, with complement-fixing IgG antibodies, leads to the generation of factors, such as anaphylatoxin and chemotactic factor, which produce an inflammatory focus. Inflammation in turn is associated with an increased transudation of serum antibodies, especially IgG. Cells are drawn to the site of inflammation, including neutrophils, macrophages, and lymphocytes. The lymphocytes include immunoglobulin-containing cells and are largely IgG. The dominance of IgG cells in inflamed tissues has been found at a number of sites such as the gingiva, synovia, urinary bladder, and kidneys. The experimental production of inflammation with repeated injections of antigens into secretory tissues of sensitized animals induces a local accumulation of IgG cells. Thus, inflammation even in secretory tissues is often characterized by a predominantly IgG response. In antigen-induced inflammations, only about 40% of the IgG cells produce specific antibody. The remaining "nonreactive" immunocytes may represent lymphocytes which are randomly seeded into the site and nonspecifically activated by blastogenic factors released from specifically stimulated cells. In addition, altered tissue or serum proteins may give rise to autoantibodies such as rheumatoid factor (anti-IgG), immunoconglutinin (anti-C3), and antitissue antibodies.

Another important function of antibody in both first- and second-line defenses may be the neutralization of toxins. For example, it is known that diphtheria antitoxin, while preventing the disease, does not influence colonization and infection by Corynebacterium diphtheriae. Although relatively little is known about antitoxic immunity in the secretory system, this could be of key importance in infections with organisms such as cholera in which the disease is caused by a toxin elaborated by the organisms in secretory tissues.

In this chapter some examples of the role of the first- and second-line mucosal defenses in specific infections will be discussed. Emphasis will be placed largely on antibody-mediated mechanisms primarily because most of the work to date on mucosal immunity has been focused in this area. However, it seems very likely that cellular (delayed-type) reactions will prove to be of great importance, and some initial studies suggesting the presence of T-cell-mediated mucosal immunity will be discussed at the end of this chapter.

VIRAL INFECTIONS

Immunity associated with local IgA antiviral antibodies

There is now rather substantial evidence that the secretory system plays an important role in infections with viruses. Figure 11-1 outlines in sche-

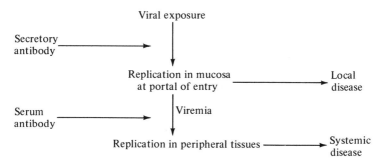

Fig. 11-1. Mechanisms of spread of viruses and postulated sites of action of serum and secretory antibody.

matic form two general patterns of viral infections. Certain viruses (e.g., myxoviruses, respiratory syncytial virus, rhinoviruses, and certain types of adenoviruses) initially colonize mucous membranes, replicate locally, and produce disease at the portal of entry, usually in the respiratory or gastrointestinal tract. In this case, there is little or no evidence of systemic dissemination, and the virus remains localized relatively superficially to the mucous membrane. Therefore, in order to interact and neutralize the virus, an antibody must act primarily at the mucous membrane level. Other viruses typified by polio, ECHO, measles, and perhaps the agent of infectious hepatitis replicate locally at the portal of entry in the mucous membrane and then undergo a phase of systemic dissemination with viremia and produce disease in peripheral organs. With this latter group of viruses, circulating antibody is effective in neutralizing the virus, probably in the blood stream and/or the interstitial fluids of susceptible tissues.

Since secretory antibody acts early in the sequence depicted in Fig. 11-1, at the site of implantation by preventing the initial colonization, it is effective in protecting against infections caused by both types of viruses. In addition, by inhibiting colonization, secretory antibody, unlike circulating antibody, may prevent the development of the carrier state.

Once an infection has become established and the virus replicates in the mucous membrane, a complex and incompletely understood sequence of events occurs which leads to elimination of the virus. Recovery from viral infections probably involves primarily second-line defenses and includes the cooperative participation of phagocytic mechanisms, serum antibody, cellular immunity, and nonimmune substances such as interferon. Although secretory antibody may also participate in the recovery process, this has not been clearly established.

The studies of Fazekas de St. Groth in the early 1950s suggested that local antibody was important in the resistance of mice to influenza virus. However, it was not until 1966 that studies in man clearly demonstrated that the titers of antibody to parainfluenza type I in nasal secretions were more closely correlated with resistance to challenge with the live virus than were the serum antibody levels. More recent studies with influenza as well as rhinovirus have also shown that secretory antibody is more closely related to protection than are the titers in the serum, the latter being largely IgG.

One of the clearest demonstrations of the importance of local immunization comes from the studies of rhinovirus infection by Chanock's group at the NIH. This virus is the most common cause of upper respiratory illness in the adult. In one study, volunteers were immunized both intranasally and parenterally with the type-13 inactivated rhinovirus. As shown in Table 11-2, both groups developed serum antibody largely of the IgG and IgM types. However, only the nasally immunized subjects developed significant titers of antibodies (primarily IgA) in their nasopharyngeal secretions. Subsequently, both groups were challenged with the live type-13 virus and only the intranasal vaccines exhibited clear-cut resistance to infection.

Further insight into the role of the secretory system in protection against viral infections has come from the extensive studies of Ogra and Karzon on immunization with polio virus. These workers measured titers of antipolio antibody in the different immunoglobulin classes in serum, nasopharyngeal fluids, and duodenal secretions. To measure antibody class, they employed a technique which involved labelling the polio virus by incorporating radioactive P^{32} into the virus during its growth phase in vitro. Utilizing the radioactive virus and anti-immunoglobulin antisera in gel diffusion, they were able to determine the class of antipolio antibody by radioautography. An example of this valuable technique, which has

Table 11-2

Rhinovirus type-13. Protection against infection by immunization by different routes.[a] Neutralizing antibodies in serum and nasal fluids following intramuscular (IM) and intranasal (IN) immunizations with rhinovirus type 13. Following immunization, volunteers were challenged with the live virus and the development of symptoms recorded. Notice that only the group which developed nasal antibody showed significant protection against challenge with the live virus.

Route of vaccination	No. in group	Geometric mean titer (reciprocal)		Illness %
		Serum	Nasal	
Intranasal	28	53.8	4.5	36
Intramuscular	11	72.5	1.5	82
Control (no vaccine)	23	4	1.3	78

[a] Data from J. C. Perkins et al., Amer. J. Epidemiology, 90:319, 1969.

recently been applied to a number of other viruses, is illustrated in Fig. 11-2. These workers found that after either parenteral (inactivated viruses) or oral immunization (live attenuated virus) serum antibody titers followed the classical sequence of IgM followed by IgG and finally a small IgA response. As illustrated in Fig. 11-3, both routes of immunization gave approximately equivalent serum titers. However, only oral immunization elicited significant titers of antibody in nasopharyngeal and gastrointestinal secretions, and the antibody in these fluids was restricted to the IgA class. Moreover, IgA antibodies in nasopharyngeal fluids (without serum antibody) could be selectively stimulated by the intranasal instillation of inactivated polio virus if the dosage of antigen used was sufficiently small. When individuals with varying titers of preexisting antibody in their nasopharyngeal secretions were challenged with the live attenuated virus, it was shown that resistance to infection was well correlated with the titers of preexisting antibody in these secretions. Figure 11-4 shows that at the particular dose of the live virus chosen they were unable to infect any subject who had a preexisting nasopharyngeal antibody titer of greater than 1 to 16. In these studies, infection was determined by measuring the amount of virus excreted in the nasopharyngeal fluids. Those individuals who had sufficient antibody were able to prevent colonization and virus excretion was not detected. If larger doses of the challenging virus were employed, resistance could be overcome.

In another series of experiments, these same workers immunized infants with double-barreled colostomies performed because of an imperforated anus. They instilled the live attenuated polio virus directly into the

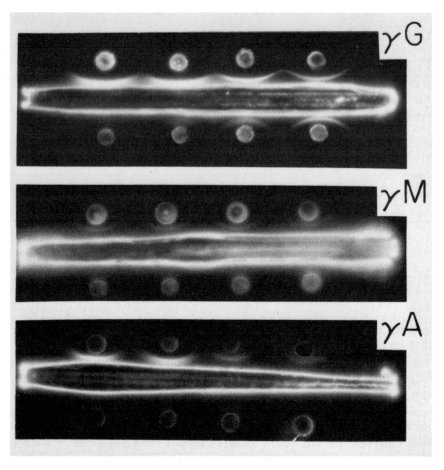

Fig. 11-2. Autoradiograph of poliovirus antibodies. The peripheral wells are filled with appropriate twofold serial dilutions of the serum or secretion to be tested, starting with the lowest dilution in the upper left-hand corner. The troughs were filled with antisera specific for IgG (γG), γM, or γA, and precipitation was allowed to occur. After washing, the central troughs were filled with 32P-labelled poliovirus, incubated, and then the slides were exposed to a photographic film. The labelled virus binds with the precipitated immunoglobulins containing the specific poliovirus antibody, thus producing a radioactive arc. (From P. L. Ogra et al., New Eng. J. Med., 279:893, 1968.)

distal colon and measured antibody titers at various sites in the GI tract. As depicted in Fig. 11-5, the highest titers of antibody, limited to the IgA class, were in the immunized segment (distal colon) with smaller titers in the proximal colon, probably as a result of spillover of infectious virus. However, no antibody was found at a really distal site in the gastrointestinal tract such as in the nasopharynx, even though high titers existed in the serum. The continuity of the bowel was subsequently surgically reestablished and the children were then fed the live polio virus orally. Viral excretion studies showed that the polio virus was able to colonize the

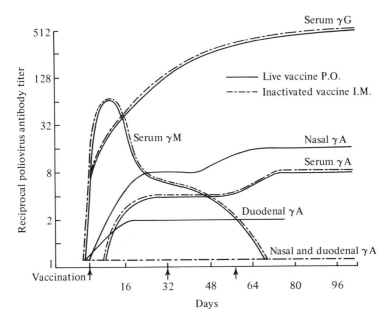

Fig. 11-3. Sequence of IgG (γG), γA, and γM antipoliovirus antibodies in serum and secretions after immunization with the inactivated virus intramuscularly and the live attenuated virus orally. (Modified from P. L. Ogra et al., *New Eng. J. Med.*, 279:893, 1968.)

nonimmune nasopharynx but that the distal colon and rectum were resistant to infection as demonstrated by the absence of virus excretion in colonic secretions. These findings clearly demonstrated that the local immunized segment, containing IgA antipolio antibodies, had developed a regional immunity which was quite independent of circulating antibody.

The participation of the regional lymphoid tissues in the nasopharynx in immunity is suggested by studies of titers of antipolio antibodies before and after removal of the tonsils and adenoids. Following tonsillectomy, preexisting antipolio antibodies in nasopharyngeal secretions dropped sharply, particularly in younger children. The effects of the tonsillectomy on preexisting antibody are less marked in older children.

Also, children who are given primary immunization following tonsillectomy have considerably lower titers than an age-matched control group. These observations suggest that the tonsil and adenoids, particularly in younger individuals, are a significant source of nasopharyngeal antibody. They also provide at least a tentative explanation for the clinical observation often quoted in the older literature that there is an increased incidence of paralytic polio following tonsillectomy.

Antibody in lower respiratory tract fluids, i.e., bronchioles and alveoli, can be stimulated by aerosol immunization using an atomizer which emits

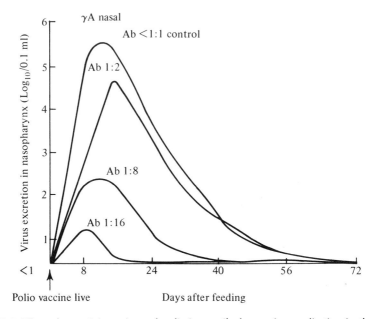

Fig. 11-4. Effect of preexisting γA nasal poliovirus antibody on virus replication in the naso-pharynx. When the preexisting antibody titers were 1:16 or greater, challenge with the live attenuated virus resulted in inhibition of implantation as evidenced by the minimal viral excre-tion in the nasopharynx. (From P. L. Ogra and D. T. Karzon, *J. Immunol.,* 102:15, 1969.)

particles of small size ($1-50\mu$). Specimens can be obtained by broncho-alveolar lavage using a cuffed bronchographic catheter. Bronchoalveolar secretions obtained from volunteers immunized with inactivated influenza virus have an IgG-IgA ratio of 2.5 to 1. This ratio is intermediate between that found for serum (5:1) and upper respiratory tract fluids such as tracheobronchial secretions and nasal washings (1:3). The observation that the ratio of influenza antibody titers in serum to bronchoalveolar fluid is high following subcutaneous immunization compared with the low ratios seen after aerosol immunization suggests that local synthesis of both IgA and IgG occurs in the lower respiratory tract.

Table 11-3 lists the viral diseases in which local production of SIgA antibodies has been demonstrated and those in which it has been shown to be important in protection.

Immunity in respiratory syncytial and measles virus infection

Infections with these viruses are considered separately since they repre-sent interesting examples of the effects of a dissociation between local and systemic immunity. Respiratory syncytial (RS) virus is the single most

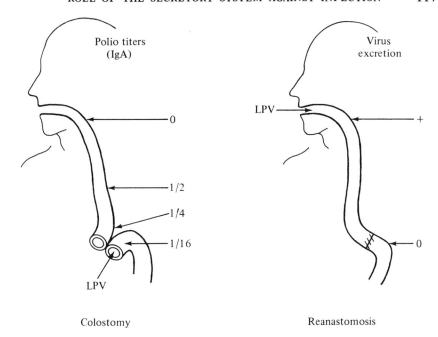

Colostomy   Reanastomosis

Fig. 11-5. Live attenuated poliovirus (LPV) was instilled into the distal opening of children with double-barreled colostomies and titers of antipoliovirus antibodies measured at different levels in the GI tract as shown on the left. After surgical reanastomosis, the live attenuated virus was fed orally and viral excretion in the nasopharynx and rectum was measured. The virus implanted (as determined by virus excretion) only in the nonimmune nasopharynx and not in the immune colon as shown in the illustration at the right.

Table 11-3

Antiviral secretory antibodies. Various viruses for which local synthesis of antibody in secretory tissues has been reported. On the right are listed those viruses in which protection against infection shows a high correlation with the titers of secretory antibody.

Local synthesis of secretory antibody (primarily IgA)	Protection against infection by secretory antibody
Polio	Polio
Influenza	Influenza
Parainfluenza	Parainfluenza
Measles	Rhinovirus
Rubella	Rubella
Respiratory syncytial	
ECHO	
Adenovirus	
Coxsackie	

frequent cause of respiratory disease in young children, particularly below the age of one year. Infections are frequently associated with bronchiolitis and pneumonia and usually occur in the first few months of life when transplacentally acquired IgG-type neutralizing antibodies derived from the mother are present in highest titer. Since infections occur most frequently when serum antibody titers are at their peak, it is apparent that serum antibody is not protective. Following immunization with an inactivated vaccine parenterally, which elevates the existing serum titers even further, immunity does not occur and in fact more serious disease often results. Maternally derived antibody and the serum antibody found following systemic immunization with the killed virus does not permeate into nasal secretions. However, natural infection does result in a significant rise in nasal fluid neutralizing activity which presumably is responsible for the immunity seen in older children and adults. Local immunization with an attenuated (cold-adapted) RS vaccine has also been successful in eliciting a nasopharyngeal antibody response, but whether this is associated with significant immunity has not yet been determined.

Why children who have been immunized systemically with the killed virus then subsequently develop a natural infection suffer a more severe illness has not been established. Speculation by several groups has suggested that, in the absence of natural mucosal immunity, the virus replicates in the lung, and if high titers of IgG-type antibodies are present in serum and pulmonary interstitial tissues, these antibodies may, on interaction with the virus, cause a local arthus-like reaction. This would, therefore, result in a type of pulmonary hypersensitivity disease induced by immune complexes. A similar explanation may apply to the peculiar and severe type of measles, often accompanied by pneumonia, which occurs in children who have been previously immunized parenterally with the inactivated measles vaccine. In these children, the local injection of measles antigen into the skin induces an arthus reaction at the injection site. Fluorescent antibody studies of the local skin lesions have demonstrated an arteritis in which measles antigen, antibody, and complement are found in the wall of the vessels. The participation of immune complexes involving viruses in the pathogenesis of disease is not without precedent in animal models. For example, in infections with the lymphocytic choriomeningitis virus in mice and in Aleutian mink disease, it has been shown that virus-antibody complexes produce a vasculitis in a manner similar to the immune complex disease (serum sickness) induced in rabbits by the injection of foreign proteins. In man, there are several reports suggesting that patients with serum hepatitis have immune complexes involving Australian antigen, and that these may induce a disseminated vasculitis resembling polyarteritis nodosa.

Although it is clear that viral-antiviral complexes can induce disease in animals, whether the unusual reactions observed following RS and measles immunization are indeed hypersensitivity phenomena resulting from immunological imbalances between the systemic and secretory systems remains to be proven. If indeed this hypothesis proves to be correct, then this is an example of a detrimental effect of immunization. It should be possible by appropriate local immunization to produce nasal fluid antibody and effective immunity, thereby avoiding these postimmunization syndromes.

Mucosal immunity associated with serum antibodies

From what has been said thus far, it seems likely that with most viruses, whether colonization of the mucous membrane will occur depends primarily upon locally produced SIgA-type antibodies. However, this does not apply to all viral infections. For example, protection against adenovirus type 4 may be mediated largely by serum antibody. Evidence for this is based on the following experiments. Adenovirus type 4 administered in enteric coated capsules to military recruits produces an asymptomatic infection in the intestinal tract and elicits serum antibodies but little or no nasopharyngeal antibody. When individuals immunized in this fashion are subsequently exposed to the epidemic form of the virus, they show significant immunity. Thus, in this situation, it appears that serum antibody is associated with significant respiratory tract immunity in the absence of locally produced antibodies. Perhaps the type-4 adenovirus penetrates deeper into the respiratory mucosa than the myxoviruses and therefore encounters serum antibody which is normally present in the submucosal interstitial fluid. Whether this is the correct explanation or immunity to this virus is mediated by some as yet unidentified factor(s) (such as cellular immunity) requires further clarification.

Another example of immunity which may be mediated by factors other than local IgA-type antibody comes from some preliminary studies on a temperature-dependent mutant of the RS virus. Volunteers with low levels of existing nasal antibody to RS virus were immunized with the mutant RS virus locally. They were found to have no change in their existing titers of either serum or secretory antibody, and the virus was not excreted in their respiratory secretions. Challenge of this group several months later with the wild-type virus showed them to be immune, whereas a control (nonimmunized) group having similar titers in their secretions became infected. Thus, immunity in this situation apparently resulted from factors (largely unknown) other than secretory antibody. This does not mean, however, that local antibodies may not be one of the important factors in resistance to the naturally acquired RS infection. Rather, these experiments point out the necessity for caution in the interpretation of experiments involving the relationship between immunity and antibody titers. For example, it is possible to show an excellent correlation between antibody titers and immunity to infection, and yet the important determinant of resistance may be another as yet unknown factor which in turn correlates with the level of secretory antibody.

Some generalizations regarding routes of immunization, drawn largely from the studies discussed above on resistance to viral infections, are summarized in Table 11-4.

Table 11-4

Summary of serum and secretory immune responses following immunization with replicating or nonreplicating viral antigens [a]

Type of antigen	Route of immunization	Systemic immune response		Secretory immune response			
				Immunized mucosal surface		Nonimmunized distant mucosal surfaces	
		Ab	CMI	Ab	CMI	Ab	CMI
Replicating (live)	Local	+	+	+	+	−	−
	Parenteral	+	+			±	−
Nonreplicating (inactivated)	Local	−	−	+	NT	−	NT
	Parenteral	+	+				

Ab   antibody
CMI   cell-mediated immunity
+   present
−   absent
NT   not tested
±   infrequently observed with few antigens

[a] Modified from P. L. Ogra and D. T. Karzon, *Pediatric Clinics of North America*, 17:385, 1970.

BACTERIAL INFECTIONS

The role of the secretory system in regulating normal bacterial flora and in providing resistance to bacterial infections is not as well understood as with viral agents. As already mentioned, a variety of specific antibacterial antibodies exist in secretions which are capable of interacting with surface antigens and coating bacteria. However, lysis, opsonization, and inhibition of growth by these antibodies have been demonstrated in only a few cases and, as discussed in Chapter 10, there is considerable controversy over the antibacterial properties of SIgA.

Local immunization against bacteria

Although there are a number of older reports, both on animals and humans, which suggest local immunity in the upper respiratory tract following infection or immunization with pneumococcus, staphylococcus, and meningococcus, these studies have not clearly documented the nature of the immune process and whether it relates to local production of secretory-type antibody. The existence of local respiratory tract immunity following parenteral immunization of military recruits with groups A and C meningococcal polysaccharide is suggested by a significant protection and reduction in nasal carriers of these organisms. Group-specific antibodies are produced in the serum following immunization, but thus far it has not been possible to correlate carrier status with nasal fluid antibody. Meningococcal meningitis is an important epidemic disease in military personnel, and future studies focusing on the protection afforded by local immunization and its relation to nasal fluid antibody will be of considerable interest.

It has been demonstrated that the topical nasopharyngeal administration of diphtheria toxoid is more efficient in eliciting nasal antitoxin than is parenteral immunization. However, as pointed out previously with the influenza system, whether systemic or local immunization is the preferred route will have to be established for each organism by field trials. Even in situations where locally synthesized mucosal antibody has been demonstrated to be of key importance in protection, this does not necessarily imply that the mucosal application of antigen will be the preferred route of immunizations.

Preliminary trials have shown that oral administration of attenuated Shigella bacillus strains results in serotype specific immunity, whereas parenteral immunization offers little or no protection from clinical infection. Agglutinating coproantibodies of the IgA and IgM classes have been identified in the feces of patients with diarrhea due to shigella. However, these antibodies have not yet been shown to play a role in immunity to or recovery from shigella infections. An attenuated (streptomycin-dependent) oral vaccine against typhoid has also been reported to be more effective than the parenteral killed vaccine, but the data are not yet extensive enough to reach final conclusions as to which vaccine is preferable.

Cholera

Immunity to cholera has been more extensively studied than to any other bacterial disease. When Vibrio cholera is ingested by a susceptible host, the organism multiplies in the small intestine, reaching numbers on the order of 10^9 organisms per ml of fluid. It is the exotoxin produced by the bacteria which results in the secretion of large volumes of isotonic fluid by the small intestinal epithelial cells, and the clinical symptoms result primarily from dehydration. Light microscopy shows little in the way of demonstrable morphological alterations in the gastrointestinal tract. Moreover, the toxin itself has not been identified in intestinal lymph or mesenteric blood in experimental cholera, suggesting that there is no significant systemic absorption. Thus, cholera appears to be a disease which is confined to the gut and does not penetrate beyond the level of the intestinal mucosa.

Immunity in cholera could result from killing or inhibition of the growth of the organism (antibacterial) or from neutralization of the toxin by antibody (antitoxin immunity). In either case, since the bacteria replicate locally in the lumen and the toxin acts superficially on the epithelial cell, it is apparent that for immune mechanisms to be effective, they must act at the mucous membrane level. There is, however, considerable controversy as to whether immunity is mediated primarily by antibody derived from serum, from locally produced (primarily IgA-type) antibodies, or both. Following natural infection or parenteral immunization with the whole-cell commercial vaccines, serum antibodies with both agglutinating and complement-dependent vibriolytic properties are detectable. The levels of these antibodies gradually diminish over the course of 6–12 months, and protection against infection is closely correlated with serum titers. Similarly, in endemic areas, resistance in nonimmunized individuals is well correlated with the level of serum antibody. However, despite the excellent correlation between immunity and serum antibody, it should not necessarily be concluded that the serum antibodies are responsible for the observed resistance to reinfection. For example, the serum titers may in turn be correlated with coproantibody which is the real determinant of immunity. Indeed, several groups have demonstrated the occurrence of cholera-specific antibodies in gastrointestinal fluids and feces from patients with active cholera as well as from stools obtained in the convalescent period. Whether these coproantibodies are locally produced or derived from serum has not been elucidated. In some reports, SIgA anticholera antibodies have been demonstrated and these would presumably be locally produced.

In human volunteers, cholera vaccine administered orally will induce a local immune response in the gastrointestinal tract with minimal serum antibody. This observation, together with the earlier studies of Burrows and his co-workers on experimental cholera in guinea pigs, showing an excellent correlation between resistance to reinfection and titers of coproantibodies, suggests that locally synthesized intestinal antibodies may contribute to immunity. Additional evidence for local gastrointestinal immunity in cholera has been obtained in animal studies employing isolated loops and slices of rabbit ileum. This work has demonstrated that the adherence and growth of the cholera organisms are markedly diminished by coproantibody, provided the intestinal cells are viable. These data have been discussed in detail in Chapter 10.

With both the whole-cell vaccine and following natural infections, there is little evidence for antitoxin immunity. However, recent work in experimental animals has shown that cholera toxoid is effective in producing immunity. One study using a cross-perfusion technique between exotoxin immunized and nonimmunized dogs has clearly shown that circulating antitoxin antibodies from the immunized animal will protect the nonimmunized bowel against local intestinal challenge with the cholera exotoxin. Although these studies by no means rule out a significant role for coproantibodies in natural and whole-cell vaccine-induced protection, they suggest that circulating antibodies may also participate in resistance to infection. In light of the above, the widespread nature of the disease, and the partial (80%) and temporary (4–6 months) protective effects of current vaccination procedures, field trials comparing different routes of immunization as well as the effectiveness of cholera toxoid will be of considerable interest.

Antibacterial activity in the urinary tract

Antibody activity has been described in urine against a variety of bacteria, viruses, and toxins, as well as antinuclear and rheumatoid factors. Antibodies have been found in both IgA and IgG and in some studies in low molecular weight (10,000–25,000) fractions. The nature of these low molecular weight substances is unknown. Precipitating activity has been reported in fractions on the order of 15,000, isolated by techniques which separate molecules according to molecular size (i.e., density gradient ultracentrifugation). Since immune precipitation is thought to require at least two antigen-combining sites, it is difficult to envisage, according to modern concepts of antibody structure, how it can occur with molecules of this size.

In human urinary tract infections, IgG antibodies directed against the infecting organisms have been found in the urine. Whether these are derived from serum or local synthesis has not been determined. In experimentally produced bladder and kidney infections, induced by directly introducing Escherichia coli into these tissues, a remarkable increase in antibody synthesis occurs in the infected bladder and kidney. The antibody is primarily of the IgG class. However, following hematogenous infections of rabbit kidneys with E. coli, more extensive renal damage occurs and local synthesis of IgA occurs in the kidney in addition to IgG. Precipitation of newly synthesized immunoglobulin fractions with antisecretory component antiserum indicates that SIgA arises later than IgG and occurs only in the most severely damaged kidneys. Since specific anti E. coli antibody cannot be detected in SIgA fractions, in contrast to the IgG, it is postulated that the late rise in IgA may represent autoantibodies formed against self-antigens released from the damaged kidneys.

The experimental studies mentioned above on the urinary tract are important since they point out very clearly that infection of a secretory organ is not always accompanied by a local SIgA antibody response. In the normal urinary bladder, there are very few lymphoid cells and in vitro organ culture studies reveal only low levels of synthesis of about equal quantities of IgG and IgA. Following infection with E. coli, there is a marked rise in synthesis essentially restricted to IgG. It would be important in future studies to determine whether the responding IgG-producing cells arose from precursors indigenous to the bladder or were derived from invaders from the circulation or both. This type of infection, therefore, is characterized primarily by the second-line defense response outlined in Table 11-1.

LOCATION OF ACTION OF MUCOSAL ANTIBODIES

From what has been said thus far, it seems likely that antibodies produced locally, and in certain cases those derived from serum, are both active in protection of the body's mucous surfaces. However, at what level these antibodies exert their protective effect is not always clear. Antibodies could interact with antigen in the submucosal area, in the epithelial cell itself, on the surface of the mucous membrane, particularly along the mucous layer lying on the surface of the epithelial cell, and/or in the lumenal contents.

Since cholera toxin is rapidly bound to the gut epithelium, and once bound cannot be neutralized by antibody, it is likely that antitoxin neutralizes the toxin on the epithelial cell surface and/or in the lumen of the gut. Similarly, in view of the superficial nature of the cholera infection, interaction with antibacterial antibodies probably occurs at the same levels.

It is known that the newborn of certain animals, such as the cow, which are agammaglobulinemic at birth, acquire antibodies from the colostrum and that these are of key importance in preventing bacterial infections. For example, as discussed in Chapter 8, newborn calves which are deprived of maternal colostrum die of E. coli septicemia within a few days of birth. This infection can be prevented by a single ingestion of colostrum. Also, transmittable gastroenteritis in swine, which is caused by a virus, is preventable by the oral ingestion of either antisera or immune milk, whereas the same materials administered parenterally are essentially ineffective. These results suggest a local action of antibody in the GI tract, probably in the lumen or on the epithelial surface.

In the human, very little if any immunoglobulin is absorbed following birth and any biological activity of the maternally derived colostral antibodies (largely SIgA) would be exerted on the epithelial surface or in the gastrointestinal lumen. Moreover, since the human newborn does not synthesize significant amounts of IgA, the externally derived colostral antibodies are essentially the only source of mucosal antibodies. It is interesting in this regard that there are several reports which suggest a lower mortality and morbidity in breast-fed compared with artificially fed infants. This is particularly striking in the reduced incidence of respiratory and gastrointestinal infections in the breast-fed group. However, since a host of complex factors are involved in mortality and morbidity statistics, it is difficult to assign an important role to colostral-derived antibodies in the reduction of infections. Perhaps the best evidence that antibodies are active after infection comes from studies which show that human newborns fed either human or cow's milk, which contains antipolio antibodies, are immune to subsequent challenge with the live attenuated polio virus administered orally. In this situation, the antibodies derived passively in the milk are apparently neutralizing the virus, either on the mucosal surface or the lumenal fluid.

LOCAL IMMUNITY IN THE LACRIMAL GLAND AND EYE

In human tears, the major immunoglobulin is 11S IgA with attached secretory component. Immunofluorescent studies of lacrimal tissues show a vast predominance of IgA cells in the interstitium surrounding the gland and secretory component in the acinar epithelial cells (see Fig. 6-3). Thus, all of the components of the secretory system appear to be present in the eye.

Experiments with several animal models have also suggested the possibility of local immunity in the eye. Guinea pig inclusion conjunctivitis is caused by a bedsonia-like organism and is similar to the acute form of human trachoma. Guinea pigs which are injected intraperitoneally with the killed organisms develop high titers of serum antibodies, but lacrimal secretion antibodies are either not present or occur in very low titers. Subsequent topical challenge of the eye with the live chlamydia results in an unmodified infection indicating a complete absence of immunity. On the other hand, if the guinea pigs are infected by dropping the live organism onto the conjunctivae, they develop an acute infection of short duration and both serum and lacrimal fluid antibodies. These animals are highly resistant to reinfection within several weeks after recovery. The serum antibodies are complement fixing and probably of the IgG class, while the lacrimal fluid antibodies do not fix complement. The latter are presumably SIgA antibodies since they react (by the indirect fluorescent antibody technique) with an antiserum made against guinea pig colostrum and absorbed with guinea pig serum. Although immunity in this system is well correlated with the appearance and titers of lacrimal fluid antibodies, the two need not be causally related. One unexplained observation is the failure of eye secretions containing high titers of antibodies derived from an immune animal to neutralize the live organism in vitro even in the presence of fresh serum as a source of alternate pathway complement components. This suggests that either lacrimal antibodies act in concert with other factors in vivo (such as cells) or that other mechanisms are of importance such as cellular immunity and/or nonimmune systems.

Human trachoma is a widespread communicable disease and the leading cause of blindness in the world. It is particularly prevalent in underdeveloped countries, and it has been estimated that one sixth of the world's population is affected. In endemic areas such as Saudi Arabia, eye secretion antibodies against this organism are present only in infected individuals. Antitrachoma antibodies in lacrimal fluids are found in all of the immunoglobulin classes, particularly IgG. This suggests that there is some transudation of serum proteins into the eye as a result of the chronic inflammation. This seems likely since transudation of serum proteins occurs particularly readily in the eye. Although spontaneous recovery sometimes occurs, chronicity often results with episodic remissions and exacerbations. In view of the chronic nature of the disease, the role of lacrimal fluid antibodies in altering the course of the infection is uncertain. It is apparent, however, that the initial infection in children is acquired early in life, usually within the first month when mucosal immunity has not yet developed. Whether the induction of local immunity, perhaps by early local immunization, would prevent the initial acquisition of an infection is an important question which is presently under study.

The most common infection of the cornea in the United States is caused by the herpes simplex virus. The disease is characterized by recurrent episodes of keratitis, sometimes leading to scarring of the cornea and permanent blindness. This infection is unusual in that persistence of the virus in the lacrimal secretions frequently occurs in the presence of IgA antibodies which are capable of neutralizing the herpes simplex virus in vitro. In the rabbit, local immunization of one eye with the dead virus produces immunity to subsequent challenge in the immunized eye only. Since the challenged animals have IgA antibody in their lacrimal secretions in the absence of detectable circulating antibodies, protection is apparently mediated by locally produced SIgA. However, once an infection becomes established in the rabbit eye, recurrences occur despite the presence of neutralizing IgA antibodies in eye secretions. This is similar to the finding in the human disease. A tentative explanation for these puzzling phenomena has been provided by the demonstration that non-neutralizing IgG class antibodies present in the tears of infected eyes prevents neutralization by IgA antibodies. A fraction of the IgG found in tears coats but does not neutralize the virus, and the live virus coated with IgG has been found in naturally infected animals. Thus, effective neutralization depends on the relative concentrations of IgA and IgG. If substantiated, the concept of a type of antibody which results in persistence of an infectious agent rather than its inactivation is extremely important and is applicable not only to herpes but to other infections such as trachoma. These antibodies would, in certain respects, be similar to blocking antibodies which occur following desensitization in allergic diseases and to the enhancing antibodies in transplant and tumor immunity.

LOCAL IMMUNITY IN THE FEMALE GENITAL TRACT

Whether the female genital tract should be considered as a part of the secretory system has been a matter of some debate. The veterinary literature contains a large number of reports suggesting that antibody titers in bovine cervico-vaginal secretions are a better indication of infection with certain microorganisms such as brucella abortus than are serum titers. Moreover, in experimental vaginal infections in animals, it is often possible to show dissociations between serum and vaginal antibody titers, suggesting either a selective concentration of serum antibody or local synthesis.

Several studies of human vaginal and cervical fluids have reported IgG:IgA ratios similar to serum. However, there are great difficulties in accurately measuring immunoglobulin in highly viscous cervical fluids. Moreover, changes in immunoglobulin content of cervical secretions have been found at different times in the menstrual cycle. More recent studies using a sensitive radioactive precipitation technique have reported a mean IgA level in cervico-vaginal fluids of 0.22 mgm/ml and IgG of 0.12 mgm/ml. A variety of conditions such as pregnancy and sterility do not alter the IgG:IgA ratio, but women over 50 have significantly more IgG in their secretions than women under 30. The elution pattern of pooled cervico-vaginal secretions on Sephadex G-200 suggested that the majority of the IgA was dimeric, and immunological studies with an anti-SC antiserum showed that the polymer IgA contained SC and was, therefore, SIgA. This finding is consistent with earlier studies showing immunofluorescent localization of SC to the cervical epithelial cells.

Early workers had shown that certain antibodies could be found in higher titers after local intravaginal immunization compared with systemic administration of the same antigen, although the classes of antibodies were not studied. More recently, the question of local synthesis of antibodies to two agents, Candida albicans and polio virus, have been investigated. Of ten cervico-vaginal samples studied for the presence of antibody to Candida albicans, eight contained IgA and three contained IgG antibodies to this organism. In all samples, 88% of the detectable anti-Candida activity was in the IgA class. Intravaginal immunization of women with a culture filtrate of C. albicans resulted in a marked rise of antibody in cervico-vaginal secretions and a lesser rise in serum. The cervico-vaginal antibody was removed by prior absorption with anti-IgA but not anti-IgG or anti-IgM. These studies, therefore, suggest local synthesis of anti-Candida antibody both during natural infection and following local application of antigen.

In most of the studies discussed above, the secretions were obtained by instilling saline into the cervical os and subsequently aspirating the fluid from the os and vaginal fornix. Thus, although the term cervico-vaginal fluids is used, the immunoglobulins in these fluids could have originated elsewhere, i.e., ovary, tubes, uterus, or even the peritoneal cavity. In a few patients who had previously had a complete hysterectomy, IgA was the predominant immunoglobulin in vaginal fluids and in these IgA must have been secreted by the vagina. The importance of separating the vaginal and uterine immune responses is illustrated by a study showing that intra-vaginal immunization with poliovirus type I results in IgA-type antibodies in cervico-vaginal fluids, while after intrauterine inoculation the antipolio response was essentially limited to IgG immunoglobulins. Intramuscular immunization produced a delayed IgG-type response in the genital fluids, the peak response being correlated with the highest IgG titers in the serum.

By means of the fluorescent antibody technique, IgA is found to be present within occasional plasma cells in the tubes and cervical submucosa. However, all of the female genital organs, especially the vagina, contain very few plasma cells. Whether the paucity of IgA plasma cells in these tissues is consistent with the concentrations of IgA found in the fluids bathing the mucosa is difficult to say. What is needed is more detailed data on the numbers of immunoglobulin-containing cells relative to the secretory rates of immunoglobulins for the various female organs.

LOCAL IMMUNITY IN DENTAL CARIES

Two types of caries have been recognized: smooth surface and pit and fissure. Caries occurring on the smooth surface of teeth have been shown to be transmissible and can be produced by monoinfection of rats with several types of streptococci, particularly Streptococcus mutans. The pit and fissure variety which occurs in an occlusal fissure or on the margin of an improperly placed filling is the more common type in man, and although the mechanisms leading to this type are more complex, several types of streptococci including S. mutans may be involved.

Caries are associated with the formation of dental plaque which consists of closely packed bacteria together with other constituents. In the center of the plaque the bacterial cells are in close approximation, and current evidence suggests that it is the acid produced by these cells which causes decalcification of the enamel and eventually caries. There are two general types of adhesions necessary in the formation of a plaque. One is between the bacteria and the surface of the tooth, and the second is between the individual bacteria composing the plaque. It can be shown that with cariogenic organisms such as S. mutans, the production of dextran by the bacterium is vital to both processes but particularly to the interbacterial adhesions. Other cariogenic streptococci such as S. salivarius are levan producers. If S. mutans is grown on glucose (rather than sucrose), it does not synthesize dextran and does not adhere to surfaces. If a small amount of dextran (on the order of 1 or 2 molecules per bacterium) is added to the culture, there is immediate clumping as the microorganisms become associated with one another. The forces involved are noncovalent and can be disrupted by urea. In the presence of sucrose, cariogenic bacteria of the S. mutans group are able to produce high molecular weight dextrans through the mediation of an enzyme system called dextran-sucrase (a glucosyl transferase) which is located on the surface membrane of the bacteria. It has been shown that antibodies to dextran-sucrase added to bacteria growing in vitro do inhibit the ability of the bacteria to make dextran, to adhere to surfaces, and to participate in the interbacterial aggregation phenomenon necessary for the formation of dental plaque.

Much of the work on immunization against caries has been done in rats monoinfected with a single type of cariogenic streptococci. Although some discordant results have been reported, several recent well-designed studies have shown that systemic as well as local immunization with whole organisms about the salivary gland does result in the production of agglutinating antibodies both in the serum and saliva, and in some instances there has been a significant reduction in the incidence of caries. In one of the most striking studies, subcutaneous immunization with killed S. mutans showed that salivary titers correlated with a striking reduction in the incidence of caries. Immunization of rats with a crude preparation of dextran-sucrase has resulted in a 40% reduction in caries compared with controls. In only one study was the class of antibodies determined and it was found that the salivary antibodies, after both systemic and local (salivary gland) immunization with S. mutans, were of the IgA type. However, the techniques employed in this study to determine the class of antibody were not entirely satisfactory, so that the results should be considered tentative, and further confirmation of the antibody class or classes is required.

In evaluating immunization studies against caries, it is important to recognize that the extent of the disease is markedly influenced by diet as well as several other factors. Caries can be eliminated if carbohydrate is withdrawn from the diet. Therefore, if a procedure is used (such as direct salivary gland immunization) which affects the animal's ability to ingest food, it may significantly influence the results. Therefore, careful controls are necessary. Another significant problem in immunization is that S. mutans, one of the major cariogenic organisms, occurs in several antigenic variants and typing of this organism has not been thoroughly investigated. Thus, it would be theoretically possible to have infections with different serotypes, and these could be constantly changing just as occurs with the serotypes of E. coli in the gastrointestinal tract. In this regard it is the type-specific protein of streptococci which is related to virulence, and this in turn can be correlated with the ability of streptococci to adhere to surfaces. Type-specific M protein antisera inhibit the absorption of strep to epithelial surfaces. The elegant work of Gibbons and his associates on the effects of antibodies on adherence of bacteria to surfaces is reviewed in Chapter 10.

Even if immunization were effective in producing high levels of salivary antibodies, there is no information in man as to whether antibody secreted into the oral cavity would be absorbed onto a dental plaque and have an effect on established caries. Perhaps more likely to be successful would be immunization of children in order to prevent the initial colonization process. Since children under one year of age do not have teeth, they do not harbor cariogenic organisms during the first year of life and, therefore, this may be a period when immunization would be effective.

The role of delayed hypersensitivity in caries has not been thoroughly investigated. This would be particularly pertinent in the pit and fissure variety since the primary lesion in this type of caries is surrounded by lymphoid cells which are abundant adjacent to the epithelium. Cellular immunity is particularly pertinent in periodontal disease and has been implicated by some workers in the pathogenesis of this disease. A discussion of this extensive area of dental research lies outside the scope of this book.

LOCAL CELLULAR IMMUNITY

In contrast to the large number of reports dealing with the humoral antibody response in secretions, only a few studies have appeared to date regarding cell-mediated immunity in secretory organs. There is, however, little question that cellular reactions of the delayed type do occur in secretory tissues such as the respiratory tract. Two significant problems make it somewhat difficult to obtain definitive studies in this area. One concerns the difficulty of isolating lymphoid cells from certain secretions, and the other, the lack of good in vitro correlates of delayed skin re-activity. Despite these problems, several good studies have appeared suggesting that the concept of local immunity can be extended to include cell-mediated immunity.

Lymphocytes can be obtained from the respiratory tract of animals by simple irrigation of the major bronchi (bronchial wash lymphocytes). The capacity of these lymphocytes to respond to a specific antigen by the liberation of macrophage inhibitory factor (MIF) is thought to be one of the better in vitro measures of cell-mediated immunity. In this test, a soluble factor liberated by sensitized lymphocytes upon contact with specific antigen has the capacity to inhibit the migration of normal guinea pig macrophages in capillary tubes. The results of experiments in which guinea pigs were immunized subcutaneously and locally by nose drops with dinitrophenylated human gammaglobulin (DNP-HGG) are sum-marized in Fig. 11-6. The spleen cells of animals which were immunized subcutaneously with DNP-HGG elaborated MIF on contact with antigen, while the bronchial wash lymphocytes exhibited little or no production of MIF. When immunization was performed by instillation of the antigen into the nose, the reverse pattern was obtained, i.e., MIF was elaborated by bronchial wash but not by splenic cells after exposure to DNP-HGG. Separation of bronchial wash lymphocytes and macrophages showed that it was the lymphocyte population (99% pure) which produced MIF and that the presence of specific anti-DNP-HGG antibody in the wash fluid did not influence their ability to produce MIF nor interfere with the assay system for MIF. Similar findings have also been reported following respira-tory tract immunization with killed influenza virus and BCG (Bacille Calmette-Guerin) in which local cell-mediated immunity has been recog-nized.

These studies demonstrate that cellular immunity in the respiratory tract can be produced independently of systemic cellular immunity. More-over, the results suggest that locally sensitized lymphocytes remain in the respiratory tract and do not migrate in significant numbers to peripheral sites such as the spleen. The origin of the sensitized bronchial wash lymphocytes has not been established, but some evidence suggests that they are produced in the lamina propria rather than the original lymph nodes.

Although there have been claims that delayed reactions occur in other secretory organs, e.g., GI tract, critical examination of these re-ports leaves some doubt as to their validity. The failure to isolate lympho-

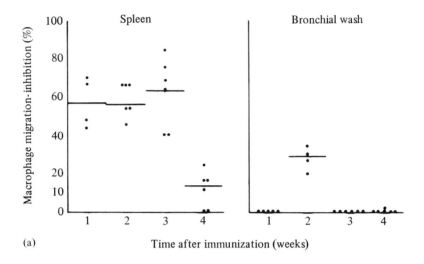

(a)   Time after immunization (weeks)

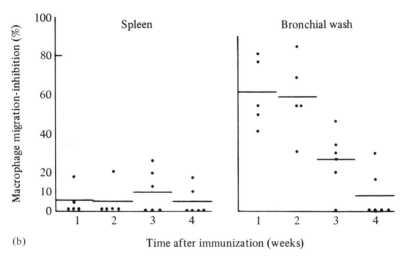

(b)   Time after immunization (weeks)

Fig. 11-6. Mean percent inhibition of macrophage migration by cells obtained from spleen and bronchial washing at various times after immunization of guinea pigs with DNP-HGG. (a) Foot pad immunization. (b) Nose drops immunization. Note that nasal immunization is more effective than the parenteral route in eliciting bronchial cellular immunity. (Data from R. H. Waldman and Christopher Henney, *J. Exp. Med.*, 134:482, 1971.)

cytes from these sites and to rule out a direct toxic effect of the antigen in contributing to the histological lesion are major drawbacks in these studies.

REFERENCES

Brandtzaeg, P.: "Local Formation and Transport of Immunoglobulins Related to the Oral Cavity," in *Host Resistance to Commensal Bacteria,* ed. by T. MacPhee, Churchill Livingstone, Edinburgh, 1972.

Chanock, R. M.: "Local Antibody and Resistance to Acute Viral Respiratory Tract Disease," in *Secretory Immunologic System,* ed. by Dayton, Small, Chanock, Kaufman, and Tomasi, U.S. Government Printing Office, Washington, 1971, p. 83.

Hanson, L. A.: "Immunoglobulins in Urines of Children with Urinary Tract Infections," in *Secretory Immunologic System,* ed. by Dayton, Small, Chanock, Kaufman, and Tomasi, U.S. Government Printing Office, Washington, 1971, p. 367.

Kaufman, H. E.: "Development of Resistance in the Eye," in *Secretory Immunologic System,* ed. by Dayton, Small, Chanock, Kaufman, and Tomasi, U.S. Government Printing Office, Washington, 1971, p. 325.

Lehmann, J. D., J. W. Smith, T. E. Miller, J. A. Barnett, and J. P. Sanford: "Local Immune Response in Experimental Pyelonephritis," *J. Clin. Invest.,* 47:2541, 1968.

Mills, J., H. L. S. Knopf, J. Van Kirk, and R. M. Chanock: "Significance of Local Respiratory Tract Antibody to Respiratory Syncytial Virus," in *Secretory Immunologic System,* ed. by Dayton, Small, Chanock, Kaufman, and Tomasi, U.S. Government Printing Office, Washington, 1971, p. 149.

Murray, E. S., L. T. Charbonnet, and A. B. MacDonald: "Immunity to Chlamydial Infections of the Eye. I. The Role of Circulatory and Secretory Antibodies in Resistance to Reinfection with Guinea Pig Inclusion Conjunctivitis," *J. Immunol.,* 110:1518, 1973.

Ogra, P. L., and D. T. Karzon: "The Role of Immunoglobulins in the Mechanism of Mucosal Immunity to Virus Infection," in *Pediatric Clinics of North America,* 17:385, 1970.

Ogra, P. L., and S. S. Ogra: "Local Antibody Response to Poliovaccine in the Human Female Genital Tract," *J. Immunol.,* 110:1307, 1973.

Reynolds, H. Y., and R. E. Thompson: "Pulmonary Host Defenses. I. Analysis of Protein and Lipids in Bronchial Secretions and Antibody Responses Following Vaccination with Pseudomonas Aeruginosa," *J. Immunol.,* 111:358, 1973.

Reynolds, H. Y., and R. E. Thompson: "Pulmonary Host Defenses. II. Interaction of Respiratory Antibodies with Pseudomonas Aeruginosa and Alveolar Macrophages," *J. Immunol.*, 111:369, 1973.

Waldman, R. H.: "Immunization Procedures," in *Clinical Concepts of Infectious Disease*, ed. by L. E. Cluff and J. E. Johnson, the Williams & Wilkens Co., Baltimore, 1972, p. 353.

Waldman, R. H., and C. S. Henney: "Cell-Mediated Immunity and Antibody Responses in the Respiratory Tract after Local and Systemic Immunization," *J. Exp. Med.*, 134:482, 1971.

Waldman, R. H., C. S. Spencer, and J. E. Johnson: "Respiratory and Systemic Cellular and Humoral Immune Responses to Influenza Virus Vaccine Administered Parenterally or by Nose Drops," *Cell. Immunol.*, 3:294, 1972.

Chapter 12

Diseases of the Secretory System

This chapter will deal with diseases which involve the secretory immune system. It is obviously beyond the scope of this monograph to discuss all of the various diseases which affect secretory organs and in which immune mechanisms may play an important role. For example, cancer of the stomach and ulcerative colitis are two common diseases involving secretory tissues in which immunity at the local level is undoubtedly important. Rather, emphasis will be placed in this chapter on diseases of the IgA system (see Table 12-1) which either affect or result from abnormalities in the secretory system.

ELEVATION OF SECRETORY IMMUNOGLOBULINS

There are few known diseases in which higher than normal levels of secretory immunoglobulins have been recognized, with the possible exception of alpha chain disease and rare cases of IgA-type myeloma which involve secretory organs. In the relatively few cases where measurements are available, there seems to be little correlation in various clinical syndromes between the level of IgA in serum and external secretions. For example, in keratoconjunctivitis sicca (Sjögrens Syndrome), characterized by dry eyes and dry mouth and lymphocytic infiltration of the salivary and lacrimal glands, the salivary IgA concentrations are usually normal and bear no direct relationship to the serum IgA levels which are often elevated. Patients with hepatic cirrhosis, rheumatoid arthritis, and anaphylactic purpura have elevated serum IgA levels which are out of proportion to the other immunoglobulins. Since IgA synthesized in secretory sites may reach the serum (see Chapter 6), it is at least theoretically possible that the secretory system is involved in some of the diseases which are characterized by high serum IgA. In anaphylactic purpura and cirrhosis, there is commonly involvement of the GI tract, and the lymphoid-plasma cell proliferation in the lamina propria could be the source of at least a part of the increased serum IgA.

Two other diseases, dermatitis herpetiformis (D.H.) and a benign

135

Table 12-1

Diseases associated with abnormalities in IgA

Increased IgA (in relation to other immunoglobulins):
 IgA myeloma
 Cirrhosis of the liver
 Alcoholic hepatitis
 Rheumatoid arthritis (especially those with high titers of rheumatoid factor)
 Systemic lupus erythematosus
 Sarcoidosis
 Anaphylactic purpura
 Wiskott-Aldrich syndrome
 Chronic lung disease (especially pneumoconiosis)

Isolated deficiency of IgA:
 Normal individuals (1 in 500–700)
 Hereditary telangiectasia (4 out of 5)
 Nontropical sprue
 Systemic lupus erythematosus [a]
 Cirrhosis of the liver [a]
 Juvenile rheumatoid arthritis [a]
 Recurrent otitis media
 Congenital rubella (transient)
 Pernicious anemia [a]

Deficiency of IgA combined with other immunoglobulin and cellular defects:
 Agammaglobulinemia-congenital, common variable (includes acquired and dysproteinemia)
 Secondary (multiple myeloma, leukemia, nephrotic syndrome, protein-losing enteropathy)
 Common variable associated with T cell deficiency

Selective deposition of IgA in tissues:
 Dermatitis herpetiformis—IgA in lumpy-bumpy deposits along dermal epidermal basement membrane
 Berger's disease—renal (mesangial) deposits of IgA

---

[a] Low frequency; actual incidence remains to be verified.

recurrent nephritis of children, are associated with immunoglobulin deposits restricted largely but not entirely to the IgA class. In D.H. there is an intensely pruritic bullous eruption associated with malabsorption syndrome. Granular "immune complex" like deposits of IgA are seen beneath the dermal-epidermal basement membrane. Some of the components of the alternative complement pathway such as properdin and C3 proactivator are also seen in active lesions. The relationship of the skin lesions to the GI disease is unknown, but the selectivity of the deposits for IgA suggests the possibility of an immune complex disease involving an antibody arising in the GI tract.

A type of recurrent nephritis characterized by episodes of hematuria frequently preceded by an upper respiratory infection has been observed in children by Berger in France. These children have relatively normal renal function and on kidney biopsy have intercapillary (mesangial) deposits of IgA, IgG, and sometimes C3 in their glomeruli. The deposition of IgA is unusual in classical acute post-streptococcal glomerulonephritis or chronic membrane proliferative glomerulonephritis. As with D.H., it has been hypothesized that complexes involving IgA antibody arise in secretory tissues and are possibly directed against ingested or inhaled antigens.

Quantitative data on immunoglobulin concentrations in secretions other than saliva in various disorders are very scanty. IgE is elevated in the nasal fluids and serum of many patients with atopic respiratory diseases such as hay fever and certain cases of asthma. Respiratory allergy such as hay fever and some cases of asthma could be considered as diseases of the secretory system probably mediated in large part by IgE. This is, however, an extensive area and will not be discussed further in this chapter. (See Chapter 10 for a brief summary of the role of IgE in allergies.)

It seems likely that, as additional studies are performed on non-vascular secretions, more deviations from normal will be found. It might be expected, for example, that normal individuals from geographic areas where sanitation is poor and infections and parasitic infestations are common would have higher concentrations of secretory immunoglobulins, as a secondary phenomenon, related to continued antigenic stimulation. In certain types of intestinal parasite diseases (e.g., capillariasis), the serum IgE level is markedly elevated, and increased numbers of IgE cells are seen in the gastrointestinal lamina propria. It would be expected in these cases that high levels of IgE would be present in gastrointestinal fluids, although this has not been demonstrated as yet.

As discussed in Chapter 2, normal serum contains small amounts of SIgA and certain diseases such as ulcerative colitis and chest infections have elevated levels of SIgA. Some of the highest concentrations have been reported in lactating women. The origin of serum SIgA is not definitely known, but presumably it represents leakage from secretory sites that tends to occur particularly when mucous surfaces are involved in inflammatory processes.

IgA *myelomas*

In the majority of patients with IgA-type myelomas, the disease is disseminated and involves a variety of bony tissues. The overall clinical syndrome is similar to that seen in the more common type IgG myelomas, and there is usually no striking predilection of IgA myelomas for secretory sites. However, in a few reported cases the initial disease appeared in secretory sites, particularly the gastrointestinal tract. For example, the author has recently seen a patient who presented initially with gastrointestinal tract disease, intraabdominal fluid, and no apparent involvement of skeletal structures. This patient had a plasma cell tumor of the small intestine and the abdominal (ascitic) fluid contained a monoclonal IgA protein which had a sedimentation coefficient of 10S with little or no 7S IgA. The absence of 7S IgA, together with the clinical picture, suggested that the origin of this protein was from GI lamina propria cells. Several similar cases have been reported in the medical literature. Why IgA myelomas almost invariably arise in the bone marrow is difficult to explain. Supposedly myelomas arise randomly by spontaneous or viral-induced mutation, and this process should occur most frequently in those sites having the greatest numbers of IgA cells. Although the marrow could be a major site of IgA synthesis, certainly a sizable proportion of the body's IgA cells are located in secretory organs and yet, as mentioned above, only a rare case arises in these sites. Perhaps the marrow is a particularly fertile area for malignant plasma cells to proliferate. Malignant cells may seed many different organs but be inhibited in their proliferation, perhaps by cellular mechanisms, except in the bone marrow.

Alpha chain disease

This disease, first described by Seligmann and co-workers in 1968, is characterized clinically by a malabsorption syndrome, frequently first diagnosed as an intestinal lymphoma. There is a diffuse lymphoplasmocytic proliferation involving the entire length of the small bowel. The serum, urine, and saliva contain a protein antigenically related to the alpha chain (H chain of IgA). This disease occurs predominantly in patients below 35 years of age and in Arabs and non-Ashkenazi Jews, although recently a few cases have also been reported in other geographic areas and ethnic groups. Alpha chain disease is probably the most common type of heavy chain disease.

The serum of patients with alpha chain disease frequently has a broad electrophoretic abnormality in the gamma-beta region rather than the typical spike-like peak seen in IgA myelomas. In about one-half the cases, the routine serum electrophoretic pattern is normal. Immunoelectrophoretic analysis shows a prominent IgA arc often extending into the β-γ regions, but the abnormal band does not react with anti-L-chain antisera. Great care must be taken to exclude myeloma since some IgA proteins, especially those with lambda light chains, do not react with L chain typing antisera. This is because of a unique conformation in which the K or λ determinants are buried or hidden. Mild reduction of disulfide linkages will often permit detection of L chains in these "untypable" proteins.

Because of the tendency of the alpha chain disease protein (αCDP) to polymerize, ultracentrifuge analysis shows marked polydispersity with the sedimentation coefficients ranging from 3–14S. The higher polymers are largely disulfide bonded and upon reduction are reduced to 3.2S. The molecular weights of the five αCDP studied thus far have varied from about 29,000 to 35,000 (polypeptide portion only). Since the polypeptide portion of the normal alpha chain has a molecular weight of about 50,000, it is obvious that these represent fragments rather than the entire alpha chain. This is also evidenced by the presence of approximately 15% carbohydrate in αCDPs, compared with about 7% for normal α chains. This suggests that the portion of the IgA molecule which is high in carbohydrate is retained in the αCDPs. Immunological analysis and the limited sequence data available both confirm the Fc nature of the alpha chain fragment. Structural analyses of the αCDP have revealed the presence of the typical hinge peptides high in proline and containing the three inter-H-chain bonds. However, the cysteine which normally links the α and L chains in IgA$_1$ proteins is absent. All 24 αCDPs which have been typed are IgA$_1$. Thus, αCDPs have a large deletion in the N terminal region of the alpha chain involving both the variable and constant region (first constant homology unit) of the Fc fragment.

It seems very likely that αCDP originates in cells of the gastrointestinal tract. Immunofluorescence and in vitro cultures of intestinal biopsies employing C^{14}-labelled amino acids have shown synthesis of the αCDP. In one reported case of a Flemish child, diffuse pulmonary and mediastinal node infiltration occurred in the absence of GI involvement. This may represent a respiratory form of the disease and again emphasizes the secretory origin of these cells. In some patients, a few alpha-chain-containing cells are found in the bone marrow, but these probably represent cells which have migrated to the marrow from their site of origin in the GI tract. It is important to recognize that in this disease, unlike μ chain disease, there is no detectable Bence Jones protein. Thus, in addition to the structural abnormality in the alpha chain, for some unknown reason, the genes controlling the L chains are not expressed. Whether these two gene defects, one involving the structure of the alpha chain and the other the synthesis of the L chain, are somehow related is at present unknown. It is possible that a regulator gene defect is present in addition to the structural gene abnormality.

A variant of alpha chain disease has been reported in a patient suffering from recurrent upper respiratory infections, who was found to have alpha chains of nearly normal molecular weight along with free L chains in his respiratory secretions. It was postulated that the defect in the alpha chain was a relatively localized one, perhaps involving a deletion of only a few amino acids including the cysteine normally linking the L and the H chains. Thus, this disease would represent an abnormality in linkage without a large deletion such as that seen in classical alpha chain disease.

DEFICIENCIES OF SECRETORY IMMUNOGLOBULINS

It is now well established that B lymphocytes possess surface immunoglobulins which are easily detected by techniques such as immunofluorescence. B cells are precursors of plasma cells, and this differentiation is initiated on contact with antigen. Some cases of agammaglobulinemia have been described in which mature plasma cells are absent but there are nearly normal numbers of B cells as determined by surface immunoglobulins. This would imply that in this group of patients there is a failure of terminal differentiation rather than a gene defect in the synthesis of immunoglobulin. This had led to the concept of blocks at various levels in the "switchover" from one cell type to another that occurs during the microevolution of antibody-forming cells. (Consult Chapter 5 for further discussion of cell differentiation.) Thus, as shown in Fig. 12-1, the various patterns of immunodeficiencies would result from blocks at certain steps, and the deficiency would involve all cells (and their products) subsequent to the block. Although this is certainly an attractive hypothesis and is consistent with the cellular patterns observed in most immunodeficiency syndromes, discrepancies still exist. For example, it is difficult to explain certain observed syndromes such as immunodeficiency with normal levels of IgG and low or absent IgA and IgM (called type II dysgammaglobulinemia in the old terminology). Although this syndrome could result from two peripheral blocks, one in IgM and the other in IgA, it may also represent some more complex and as yet unknown alternative mechanism which will require modification of the simplified scheme depicted in Fig. 12-1.

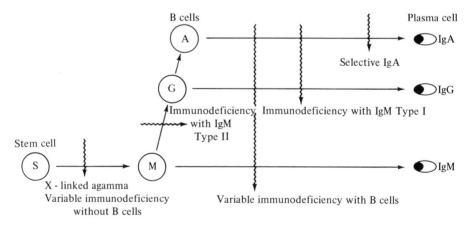

Fig. 12-1. Postulated locations of defects in the various immune deficiency syndromes. Sequential development of immunocytes from stem cells to IgM and then IgG and IgA. Sites of blocks indicated by arrows. (Modified from M. D. Cooper and A. R. Lawton, *Am. J. Pathol.,* 69:513, 1972).

Agammaglobulinemia

Patients with congenital and acquired agammaglobulinemias who have a severe deficiency of all of the major immunoglobulin classes also have a concomitant deficiency in secretory immunoglobulins. These patients usually suffer from recurrent pyogenic infections, particularly of the respiratory tract. In some patients with acquired hypogammaglobulinemias there is an associated defect in cellular immunity, and infections with intracellular organisms such as tuberculosis and parasitic fungi are also common. Because of the complex nature of the immune abnormalities in these patients, involving both serum and secretory immunoglobulins and, in certain cases, cell-mediated immunity, it is difficult to evaluate the specific role played by the secretory system in the pathogenesis of these infections.

Certain patients with the common variable immunodeficiency syndromes, particularly those involving a deficiency of IgA and IgM, often have diarrhea and malabsorption syndrome. In most cases the intestinal mucosa shows flattened villi similar to that seen in classical sprue, and immunofluorescence reveals decreased numbers or absence of plasma cells in the lamina propria. Occasionally a patient will have abundant plasma cells which by immunofluorescence are IgG, reflecting the predominance of IgG in the serum. Some patients have nodular accumulations of lymphocytes which are large enough to be visualized by roentgenographic examination of the small intestine. It has been suggested that the various clinical syndromes result, at least in part, from a deficiency of IgA at the mucous surface, and this in turn leads to an increased susceptibility to intestinal as well as respiratory infections.

The majority of patients with acquired hypogammaglobulinemia and steatorrhea harbor Giardia lamblia. This is a protozoan organism which is well known as a cause of traveler's diarrhea. Most otherwise normal individuals infected with this organism do not have malabsorption, although a few patients have more prolonged diarrhea and clinical and chemical evidence of malabsorption and a sprue-like pattern on intestinal biopsy. These patients respond rapidly to specific therapy (i.e., atabrine). One report suggests that normal individuals who acquire acute giardia infections (without malabsorption) have a partial defect in their secretory system. The evidence for this statement was the finding that duodenal aspirates of ten cases of acute giardiasis several months after eradication of the parasite with quinacrine had IgA concentrations which were about half that of normal controls. Serum IgA concentrations were normal. This study, if substantiated, has important implications in terms of partial defects restricted to the secretory system as a predisposing factor to infection. It may be that the potential for giardia-induced malabsorption is greater in hypogammaglobulinemia than in normal individuals, and that giardia is responsible for a significant portion of the cases of malabsorption associated with hypogammaglobulinemia. Alternatively, the high frequency of infection with this organism may be a secondary manifestation of the immune disorder, and the parasite itself is not primarily responsible for the malabsorption, although it could be an additional contributing factor. In either case, it is important to treat giardiasis when it is present in a symptomatic patient, since some patients will respond dramatically with a return of the villus architecture to normal.

In the majority of patients, the failure to culture specific organisms (other than giardia) and the lack of response to various antibiotics is against infection as a primary etiological agent. It is also pertinent in this regard that patients with congenital agammaglobulinemia and severe deficiencies of secretory immunoglobulins only rarely have diarrheal syndromes and malabsorption as a major clinical problem. In general, patients with hypogammaglobulinemic sprue respond poorly to a gluten-free diet which has been so successful in the treatment of patients with classical sprue. In a few cases, however, a good clinical response to gluten restriction has been recorded.

Selective deficiency of IgA

Studies of large populations suggest that an isolated deficiency of serum IgA occurs in about one of 500–700 individuals. A practical point which could influence the observed incidence in surveys is the type of antisera employed to quantitate IgA. If goat anti-human IgA is used, the number of IgA-deficient sera may be significantly underestimated. This is because 30–40% of IgA-deficient sera contain IgG-type antibodies which will precipitate goat serum proteins. This is a cross-reaction with goat serum proteins (see Chapter 10 for discussion). Usually only the three major classes of immunoglobulins (IgG, IgA, and IgM) are measured and, therefore, it is not certain that the deficiency is selective for IgA. However, there is no question that some completely asymptomatic individuals are selectively deficient in IgA and have normal levels of IgG, IgM, IgD, and IgE as well as intact cellular immunity. Thus, IgA deficiency when it is truly selective need not be associated with recurrent infections or other diseases. Asymptomatic individuals who have no serum IgA, when tested by a sensitive technique such as complement fixation or electroimmunodiffusion, invariably have an associated absence of IgA in their secretions, but IgA is replaced by IgM and IgG. This replacement phenomenon, along with normal cellular immunity and nonimmunological defense mechanisms, may explain why these individuals are asymptomatic.

There have been several reports of patients with a serum IgA deficiency who have IgA in their secretions and normal numbers of IgA cells in their gut lamina propria. This type of discrepancy, in the author's experience, is not found when IgA is truly absent from serum. We have observed several patients with very low serum IgA's (about $\frac{1}{10}$ to $\frac{1}{20}$ of normal) who have essentially normal numbers of cells containing IgA in their gastrointestinal tracts. It would be important to carefully study those patients who have been reported to have an absence of serum IgA and yet a normal complement of IgA-containing plasma cells in secretory sites. If such patients do indeed exist, it is possible that they could have a defect similar to that described in irradiated mice (see Chapter 6) in which the IgA produced in the submucosal area is preferentially shunted into the lumen of the bowel. Alternatively, the presence of high titers of circulating anti-IgA antibodies (see below) could prevent access of IgA from the lamina propria to serum. An analogous situation has been produced in mice by the administration of anti-mouse-IgA from birth to early adulthood. These animals have no detectable circulating IgA, and an absence of IgA cells in the spleen, but essentially normal numbers of IgA cells in the gut.

As discussed earlier in this chapter and in Chapter 5, plasma cells secreting IgA develop from B cells on contact with antigen. Several studies have reported that selective IgA-deficient patients almost invariably have normal numbers of B lymphocytes bearing surface IgA. This includes patients with sporadic and familial forms as well as those associated with hereditary telangiectasia and congenital rubella. This is schematically illustrated in Fig. 12-1. All patients with a selective IgA deficiency seem to show a common defect involving the failure of IgA-B cells to differentiate into plasma cells secreting IgA. Why antigen does not trigger the B cell is presently unknown. The observation that anti-IgA stimulates blast transformation in lymphocyte cultures of IgA-deficient patients to the same extent as in normal control cultures suggests that the IgA-B lymphocytes are not defective in the cellular mechanisms needed for transformation. In many cases, IgA deficiency is associated with T cell defects, and there is some evidence that IgA antibody responses are more thymic-dependent than those in other classes, particularly IgM. This suggests the possibility that, in certain patients, the defect in differentiation may result from a lack of helper T cell function rather than some abnormality in the B cells themselves. In other cases, T cell function appears to be intact and other unknown mechanisms are responsible. One possibility presently under investigation is excess numbers of suppressor T cells.

Although, as discussed above, IgA deficiency occurs in asymptomatic individuals, taken as a group, individuals who selectively lack IgA have a high association with various diseases. Most frequent is a history of recurrent infections, although allergic disorders such as urticaria, eczema, or asthma are also common. We have found that children with recurrent ear infections have a higher than normal incidence of IgA deficiency. Autoimmune phenomena, malabsorption, and cancer also seem to occur with increased frequency. Most cases of hereditary telangiectasia are associated with IgA deficiency. In some patients, especially in hereditary telangiectasia, there is an associated IgE deficiency, and a sizable proportion also have defects in cellular immunity. It seems likely that IgA deficiency, when associated with partial or severe defects in cellular immunity, is almost always clinically symptomatic. These relationships are summarized in Fig. 12-2.

Most cases of selective IgA deficiency, except those associated with ataxic telangiectasia, occur sporadically, and there is no evidence of a well-defined pattern of inheritance. For example, in studying siblings of patients with IgA deficiency, the incidence of abnormalities in serum immuno-globulins is far less than the 25% expected for a recessive disorder. How-

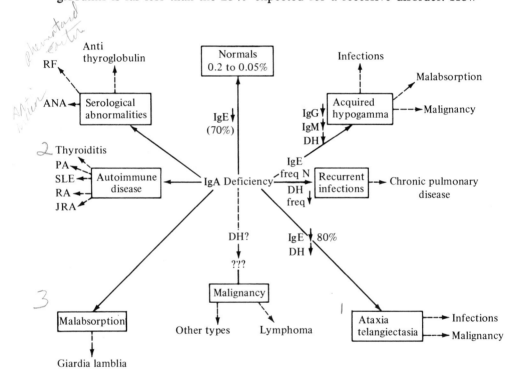

DH = Delayed hypersensitivity
RA = Rheumatoid arthritis
JRA = Juvenile rheumatoid arthritis
PA = Pernicious anemia
SLE = Systemic Lupus Erythematosus

Fig. 12-2. Interrelationships in IgA deficiency. Clinical syndromes and diseases associated with a deficiency of IgA.

ever, the pattern of inheritance does rarely suggest an autosomal recessive or even dominant disorder. In some cases, there is an association in families between non-sex-linked agammaglobulinemia and IgA deficiency, but even here there is no clear pattern of inheritance.

Although chromosome abnormalities have been reported in IgA deficiency, especially a partial deletion of chromosome 18, this is by no means a consistent finding and the relationship may be fortuitous. Many patients with choromosome 18 abnormalities do not have an IgA deficiency, and most IgA deficient patients have no chromosomal abnormalities.

ASSOCIATIONS WITH OTHER DISEASES

Association with hereditary ataxic telangiectasia

Ataxic telangiectasia is a rare recessive disorder characterized clinically by cerebella ataxia, vascular telangiectasia, and recurrent infections. Approximately 75% of these patients have an associated partial or complete deficiency of IgA, and almost all of them have defects in delayed hypersensitivity. The latter probably results from a thymic abnormality since autopsy shows an embryonic thymus. IgE deficiency also occurs in about 75% of these patients. Because of the complex nature of the immune abnormalities involving several immunoglobulins (IgE and IgA) as well as cellular deficiencies, it is dangerous to attribute too much significance to any one factor as being responsible for the increased susceptibility to infection. The relationship of the IgA and IgE deficiencies to the neurological disease is unknown. It seems unlikely that the immunoglobulin deficiencies are responsible for the central nervous system manifestation, since some patients with neurological disease have normal or elevated IgA and IgE levels. The author has seen two brothers with equivalent degrees of neurological involvement; one had an absence of IgA, and the other had normal levels. Patients with this disease usually die before age 25 of infection or malignancy. Although various types of malignancies occur, lymphoma is most common.

A selective deficiency of secretory IgA with normal levels of serum IgA, perhaps associated with defects in secretory component, has been noted by the author in several patients having recurrent infections but this syndrome has not yet been well documented.

Association with autoimmunity and malignancy

A relationship between IgA deficiency and autoimmunity has been suggested on the basis of clinical associations. Diseases which have been reported to be associated with IgA deficiency include a long list of so-called "autoimmune" disorders: Systemic lupus erythematosus (SLE), dermatomyositis, thrombocytopenic purpura, thyroiditis, Addison's disease, rheumatoid arthritis, hepatitis and chronic liver disease, regional enteritis, ulcerative colitis, nephritis, Sjögren's syndrome, pulmonary hemosiderosis, and pernicious anemia. Of this group, the most common associations are with rheumatoid arthritis, pernicious anemia, thyroiditis, and SLE, although the majority of patients with these diseases have normal or elevated IgA levels. In addition, serological abnormalities such as rheumatoid factor, antinuclear factor, and antithyroid antibodies have been noted with increased frequency in IgA-deficient patients and, in some cases, their families. Although the relationship of the IgA deficiency to many of the individual disorders mentioned above is far from established, as a group the associations are impressive. One mechanism whereby a deficiency of IgA (frequently with an associated cellular defect) might be associated with multiple clinical syndromes is through an increased susceptibility to infection with different viruses which might, in turn, cause the various diseases. Also, as discussed in Chapter 10, IgA-deficient patients have a high incidence of antibodies to milk proteins, and absorption of ingested antigens may be excessive. Continued absorption over a prolonged period of time could lead to an immune complex disease such as SLE. Another possible mechanism involves the formation of antibodies to exogenously absorbed antigens that cross-react with endogenous antigens such as those of the thyroid, stomach, and joints. This would be analogous to the formation of antibodies to streptococci which cross-react with heart muscle in rheumatic fever.

Statements have been made in the literature that patients with various immunological deficiencies have an incidence of malignancy approximately 10,000 times that of the general population. In hereditary telangiectasia, about 10–15% of the patients develop malignancies but, as indicated above, defects in delayed hypersensitivity are also present and these are known to increase susceptibility to malignancy. Therefore, no conclusions can be drawn regarding the effect of IgA deficiency per se on malignancy. It is reasonable that, if malignancies such as lymphomas are initiated by oncogenic viruses whose portal of entry involves the secretory system, deficiencies of this system could increase susceptibility to malignancy.

Association with malabsorption

Selective IgA deficiency seems to be associated with a malabsorption syndrome, although the incidence of malabsorption in IgA deficiency is not nearly as great as it is in acquired agammaglobulinemia. Moreover, some patients who present initially as a more-or-less selective IgA deficiency subsequently develop partial deficiencies of other immunoglobulins, particularly IgG, and/or have relatives with hypogammaglobulinemia. These patients may therefore have acquired agammaglobulinemia, and current evidence suggests that this is probably distinct from selective IgA deficiency. However, a few well-documented cases of IgA deficiency which have remained selective over several years have been associated with steatorrhea and have intestinal biopsies typical of nontropical sprue. IgA deficiency occurs in about one of every fifty patients with nontropical sprue. This is about twelve times the incidence in the normal population. Nodular lymphoid hyperplasia has been noted in several cases, and Giardia lamblia infestation is frequently found, as it is in acquired hypogammaglobulinemia. Some patients respond to a gluten-free diet and a few good responses to a combination of plasma infusion and antibiotics have been noted. The role of giardia in this diesase has not been thoroughly evaluated.

Most patients with classical nontropical sprue (with normal IgA) are sensitive to gluten since they respond to a gluten-free diet. After oral challenge with gluten, intestinal biopsies from these patients show a two- to fivefold increase in IgA and IgM synthesis, most of which is antigluten antibody. It has been postulated that a local antigen-antibody reaction is somehow responsible for the gluten hypersensitivity. In IgA-deficient patients with malabsorption, the IgA-type antigluten antibodies could be replaced by IgM. However, it is difficult to explain on this basis the occasional patient with agammaglobulinemia who responds to gluten withdrawal since most agammaglobulinemic patients have few, if any, plasma cells in their intestinal lamina propria. It is possible that those rare gluten-sensitive enteropathies associated with agammaglobulinemia are among the few that have intestinal plasma cells (usually IgG). More studies correlating clinical response to gluten with intestinal synthesis of immunoglobulins in agammaglobulinemic patients are needed.

ANTIBODIES TO IgA IN HUMAN SERA

Antibodies to IgA in human sera were first described in patients with ataxia telangiectasia when two patients with this disease were shown to have an excessively rapid catabolism of infused normal IgA. Subsequently, it was demonstrated that this resulted from the presence of circulating IgA antibodies which were causing immune elimination of the infused IgA. Approximately 40% of individuals with a selective deficiency of IgA have anti-IgA antibodies usually of the IgG class. These can be demonstrated by several techniques, including passive hemagglutination of red cells coated with myeloma IgA. Three types of antibody specificities have been described: those which react with all IgA myelomas and are, therefore, class-specific; a second type which shows subclass specificity reacting with either

IgA$_1$ or IgA$_2$ subgroups; and a third variety which has an even more restricted specificity reacting only with certain genetic markers on IgA. Thus far, all antibodies showing genetic specificity are directed against the AM2(+) genetic marker associated with the IgA$_2$ subclass (see Chapter 3). The class-specific antibodies are restricted to patients with selective IgA deficiency, and they seem to be primarily responsible for the severe transfusion reaction encountered in IgA-deficient patients infused with products containing IgA. The antibodies with more limited specificities are found in both IgA-deficient sera and in sera with normal IgA levels. These antibodies probably arise from isoimmunization by foreign allotypes. However, the majority of individuals, both normal and IgA-deficient, who have anti-IgA have not, to their knowledge, received injections which might have contained IgA. One possibility is that maternal isoimmunization occurred as a result of the leakage of small amounts of IgA synthesized in utero by the fetus across the placenta. It is at least theoretically possible in this situation that anti-IgA antibodies of the IgG type of maternal origin subsequently suppressed fetal IgA synthesis in a manner analogous to allotype suppression in animals. Allotype suppression refers to the long-term suppression of a particular immunoglobulin allotype in the newborn of mothers immunized during pregnancy with a paternal allotype. In our laboratory, experiments with infused anti-IgA in mice have demonstrated that a long-term depression of serum IgA can be achieved although, interestingly, the secretory system still contains sizable numbers of IgA plasma cells.

Another type of antibody to IgA has been described in about 30% of normal human sera. These naturally occurring antibodies are reactive with antigenic determinants on the F(ab)$_2$ fragment revealed by pepsin digestion of IgA. These antibodies occur in low titer, are not reactive with native IgA, and are not associated with transfusion reactions. They show no subgroup or genetic specificity, and there is no known correlation between these antibodies and specific diseases.

TREATMENT OF IgA DEFICIENCY

The presence of anti-IgA antibodies in the sera of IgA-deficient patients has important implications in the management of these patients. Anaphylactic transfusion reactions characterized by flushing, abdominal pain, vomiting, diarrhea, fever, and sometimes bronchospasm have been reported in transfused IgA-deficient patients. These reactions are immediate in onset and may occur after as little as 10 cc of blood has been administered. It has been clearly shown that these reactions are due to the patient's anti-IgA reacting with infused IgA.

If multiple infections are a clinical problem in the IgA-deficient patient, treatment should consist primarily of antibiotics and *not* commercial gammaglobulin preparations, since these preparations contain small but antigenically significant amounts of IgA. Even if it were possible to infuse large amounts of IgA without incident, it is doubtful that it would reach mucous membranes in significant amounts. Moreover, if the patient does not initially have anti-IgA antibodies, the likelihood of producing them and the risk of anaphylactic reactions on subsequent administration of blood products are substantial. For these reasons, the author feels that gammaglobulin or plasma infusions are contraindicated in the treatment of selective IgA deficiency. If these patients must be transfused (i.e., postoperatively), they should be given IgA-deficient blood or carefully washed cells or frozen diglycerolized erythrocytes. In elective surgical procedures, the patient can be plasmapheresed preoperatively and the autologous plasma used, if necessary, postoperatively along with washed or preferably frozen diglycerolized cells. Cells should be administered very slowly and discontinued at the earliest sign of a reaction.

Despite what has been said above, many patients with IgA deficiency have been repeatedly given gammaglobulin or plasma infusions without reactions. In a few isolated patients, associated arthritis or malabsorption syndrome have been reported to respond to plasma infusions. However, no control studies on the effect of plasma infusions or IgA-rich preparations on recurrent infections or other associated manifestations have been reported, and because of the risk of a transfusion reaction, the author believes such studies are contraindicated at the present time. Why some patients and not others can tolerate multiple plasma infusions without reaction is unclear. It may be that those who do tolerate transfusions are not completely deficient in IgA, and these individuals would not be expected to produce anti-IgA. Also, it is at least theoretically possible that, if infusions were given in large amounts and repeatedly, tolerance to IgA could develop.

REFERENCES

Ammann, A. J., and R. Hong: "Selective IgA Deficiency Presentation of 30 Cases and a Review of the Literature," *Medicine,* 50:223, 1971.

Good, R.: "Relations Between Immunity and Malignancy," *Proc. Nat. Acad. Sci.,* 69:1026, 1972.

Kunkel, H. G., L. M. Jerry, and W. K. Smith: "Selective Deficiency of γA Globulines; Occurrence of γA Antibodies and Their Specificities," *Proc. 6th Int. Immunopath. Symp.,* in *Immunopathology,* ed. by P. A. Miescher, Grune and Stratton, New York, 1972, p. 51.

Lawton, A. R., S. A. Royal, K. S. Self, and M. D. Cooper: "IgA Determinants on B-Lymphocytes in Patients with Deficiency of Circulating IgA," *J. Lab. Clin. Med.,* 80:26, 1972.

McFarlin, D. E., W. Strober, and T. A. Waldmann: "Ataxia-Telangiectasia," *Medicine,* 51:281, 1972.

Mattioli, C. A., and T. B. Tomasi: "Disorders of Immunoglobulin Synthesis," in *Principles of Immunology,* ed. by N. R. Rose, F. Milgrom, and C. J. van Oss, The Macmillan Company, New York, 1973, p. 333.

Seligmann, M., M. Mihaesco, and B. Frangione: "Studies on Alpha Chain Disease," *Ann. N.Y. Acad. Sci.,* 190:487, 1971.

Index

151